PRAISE FOR DR. ANIK ST. MARTIN AND *SKIN ON FIRE*

“An exceptionally helpful book for anyone with psoriasis, filled with well-researched and clearly presented information. Certain to become a literary classic in the ‘food as medicine’ genre, *Skin on Fire* provides a valuable roadmap to health that addresses the underlying causes of autoimmunity. You’ll want to buy two copies of this impactful book—one to keep and one to gift. It’s that good.”
DERENDA RICHARDSON, N.D.

“Implementing gut-healing supplements and making anti-inflammatory switches to my diet has helped immensely with my scalp psoriasis flareups!”

ELLA CHENAULT

“I began seeing Dr. Anik due to health conditions such as lupus, psoriasis, and GERD. She offered me supplements and a five-day fasting-mimicking diet to begin the healing process and reset my body for a fresh start. Thanks to her guidance and expertise, this has allowed me to feel more rested, gave me a clearer mental state of mind, and improved my digestion and skin conditions. This journey has been life changing.”
DUANE FARWELL

“As a runner and former triathlete, now in my fifties, I’ve benefited tremendously from Dr. Anik St. Martin’s guidance. She introduced me to fasting-mimicking practices that transformed my relationship with food—shifting my focus toward mindful, intentional eating that fuels both my performance and my overall well-being."

KATHRYN ACORDA HARLAN

"My husband and I brought our two-year-old daughter to Dr. Anik when we noticed that she was dealing with a nagging rash. It started out in her inner elbows and quickly spread to her to neck, chest, back, and knees. We got rid of allergens and tried every cream out there, spending hundreds of dollars. Dr. Anik explained that healing needs to start from within. We followed her advice and soon, after a couple months, we saw our little girl's rash disappearing. It's been half a year and her skin is like brand new, as it was when she was born."

ASHLEY YANT

"What makes this book stand out is that Dr. Anik St. Martin combines her real-life experience as both a sufferer *and* a practicing chiropractor with solid research on the root causes of autoimmunity. She delivers a deeply personal, no-BS account of her own healing journey—from the shame and helplessness of living with visible plaques to the freedom of clear skin she's maintained for years. She doesn't just criticize conventional treatments, she offers us a clear, actionable natural plan we can follow instead of using them."

ALICIA WINGREN

SKIN ON FIRE

HEALING PSORIASIS NATURALLY

Anik St. Martin, D.C., DACCP

Anik St. Martin Books
LONGVIEW, WASHINGTON

Disclaimer: This publication contains the opinions and ideas of its author. It is intended to provide helpful and informative material on the subjects addressed in the publication. It is sold with the understanding that the author and publisher are not engaged in rendering medical, health, or any other kind of personal professional services in the book. The reader should consult his or her medical, health, or other competent professional before adopting any of the suggestions in this book or drawing inferences from it.

The author and publisher specifically disclaim responsibility for any liability, loss, or risk, personal or otherwise, which is incurred as a consequence, directly or indirectly, of the use or application of any of the contents of this book.

Anik St. Martin/Anik St. Martin Books
www.anikstmartin.com/skinonfire
anik@comcast.net

Special discounts are available on quantity purchases by corporations, associations, and others. For details, contact the author at the address above.

Library of Congress Control Number 2026912383

Skin on Fire / Anik St. Martin —first edition

ISBN 979-8-9952726-0-1 (paperback)
ISBN 979-8-9952726-2-5 (epub ebook)

To my husband, Darin

CONTENTS

INTRODUCTION

Wearing the fiery red symptoms of an autoimmune illness on one's skin for the whole world to see is a painful experience that people with psoriasis share. Those of us who have lived with psoriasis understand the feeling of not having control over our bodies, of being at the mercy of what we look and feel like when we wake up in the morning. We're afraid to open our eyes because of possible further spread—more redness, more flaking, more cracking. And although we realize that the geography of our skin is large, the patches can seem to occupy most of the space. But even when the patches of psoriasis plaques are small in comparison, we often feel stuck and frustrated. Although we may think, *It couldn't possibly get any worse,* we know very well that it can, because it has. Over time, we learn to brace ourselves for that inevitability.

Despite outward appearances, psoriasis isn't a skin problem; it is an autoimmune problem that expresses itself through the skin. There's a difference. According to WebMD, "Autoimmune diseases result when your immune system is overactive, causing it to attack and damage your body's own tissues."[1]

Autoimmune illnesses don't simply occur without causes. Experiencing one is not just the "luck of the draw." Psoriasis is not the result of random happenstance; and despite what we are told, it is *not* idiopathic—not mysterious in origin. Typically, by the time psoriasis begins to express itself visibly, a person's body has been trying to adapt to various immune problems. Most likely, it has expressed other symptoms far before the first skin lesion appears.

Our bodies do not randomly begin to make errors. We *can* figure out what the origins of our psoriasis are if we study our personal histories, looking for clues.

Conditions associated with a compromised immune system might include problems with our tonsils, adenoids, and menstruation. Typically, chronic health problems like asthma, allergies, constipation, irritable bowel syndrome (IBS), Raynaud's syndrome, sinus infections, ear infections, and such also frequently precede the onset of psoriasis.

An exception to the slow, chronic buildup toward the development of psoriasis could be in the event of a sudden, physically traumatic insult or injury, like a chemical exposure, or an emotionally traumatic event that overstimulates the nervous system.

In my case, the causes were both chronic buildup of sensitivity to certain foods and sudden insult. I had my adenoids removed when I was two because I couldn't breathe through my nose. Adenoids are small glands behind the nasal cavity that help the body fight germs. Mine must have been swollen. Even by that age, I was having immunity problems.

Why might my immune system have been compromised as a toddler? Because of what happened to me as an infant. My mother's microbiome—the collection of microbes in her gut and vagina that I inherited during birth—may have been imbalanced. Also, by the time I was five days old, in order to help little five-pound-preemie me stay asleep through the night without needing to be fed, the pediatrician recommended that my parents put processed rice cereal in my nighttime bottle of formula. Infant digestive systems aren't mature enough to digest grain and the cascade of inflammation just continued from there.

It has since been established that the early introduction of grain can damage the intestinal lining's tight junctions, which eventually results in leaky gut syndrome and autoimmunity. For these and other reasons, the American Academy of Pediatrics no longer recommends this practice.[2]

Over years of study, practice, and healing my own body, I've found that psoriasis most commonly develops from five overlapping root causes. These are:

- **Immune disruption.** Immune system damage can start early, with in-utero stressors and traumas at birth. Further damage can occur with the use of specific drugs like steroids and antibiotics in childhood and with the many other lifelong immune system disruptors like environmental pollutants and underlying infections. When autoimmunity is allowed to go unaddressed, the resultant plethora of medical treatments only mask the body's "check engine light."

- **Inflammation.** Psoriasis is an inflammatory condition. The causes, both sudden and chronic, of inflammatory damage can be handled successfully—but only once they've been precisely identified.
- **Trauma and stress.** Emotional trauma and stress are often the elephant in the room when it comes to psoriasis—and the only way to eat an elephant is one bite at a time. With biohacking and altering lifestyle habits, you can engender real, lasting healing. It is the habit change that restores health.
- **Toxicity.** For years, I didn't realize that I was perpetuating toxicity in my body through my choice of food and beverages, cleaning products, skin care products, and medications. I had to study my responses to different substances and replace the ones that triggered symptoms. Once I did this kind of work, healing became very simple. The same pragmatic experimentation can reduce toxicity in anyone's body. For psoriasis sufferers, toxicity is a big trigger.
- **Gut dysbiosis.** The digestive system is the main system that needs to be healed to end psoriasis. All healing starts in the gut. Once I created a step-by-step gut healing system for myself, everything else fell into place. In this book, I will describe the steps to take to heal your gut.

The worst part of psoriasis is living at its mercy. For years, I lived this narrative—and recent statistics tell me that 125 million other people are sharing in the same harsh reality of psoriasis that I did—but I also know that healing is possible. Twenty years ago, I discovered a new way of healing from psoriasis through trial and error. From this, I know with certainty that there is hope for you. Smooth, silky, blemish-free skin is possible to attain and maintain. Now I have gratitude every day for my healthy, clear skin and, as a professional chiropractor, I have guided many patients through the process necessary to duplicate these results.

Why Conventional Medical Treatment Falls Short

The healing I personally experienced was not instantaneous. First, I tried all the steroids, lotions, potions, tars, vitamin D creams, chemotherapy drugs, and everything else under the sun that people with psoriasis commonly use when trying to get relief from their symptoms, except for biological drugs, and none of them worked for me. In fact, the treatments I tried mostly seemed to make my condition worse.

If we handle just the skin (treating it from the outside in with topical creams), or both the skin inflammation and replication (treating it from the inside out with antimetabolite drugs, like methotrexate, or biologics, like Tremfya), we may have relieved the symptoms temporarily but still have done nothing to address the root cause of the autoimmunity. Therefore, it's just a matter of time before we layer on another immune diagnosis, like Hashimoto's disease, systemic lupus erythematosus (SLE), rheumatoid arthritis, or cancer.

The Natural Healing Path

We are all born with an inherent ability to heal. Self-healing is one of the human body's most important innate gifts. Until the moment we are dead in the cold ground, our bodies are constantly trying to find a way to overcome defects and damage to keep us alive and functioning. This propensity toward survival and health is fundamental and undeniable. Healing *is* our natural default.

If this capacity was a lamp you owned and you have psoriasis, you might say that the light of its bulb has become dimmed—and if your symptoms are severe, maybe your body cannot even flip the lamp's "on" switch anymore. With too great a load put on our ability to adapt, the process by which we express health becomes faulty. Fortunately, it is our destiny to move toward health, and that is what I learned to do to return to a healing state.

Healing Psoriasis Naturally is a step-by-step guide to the daily routines and practices I have found truly work. Through experience, and sometimes despite myself, I developed this tried-and-true protocol, which I've used time and time again to help people from all walks of life, including in my own private chiropractic practice over the past twenty-four years.

I wish I'd had this information available to me when I was twenty-five years old, but I am filled with gratitude that today, at fifty years old, I have the opportunity to share it with you. The topic of healing psoriasis naturally is close to my heart because it is rooted in my own journey of physical, mental, and emotional healing. But this book also presents objective facts, as it is a product of three decades of thorough study of the literature describing the most advanced scientific research on gut health, autoimmunity, nutrition, and how to successfully bring it to the kitchen, and neurobiology.

In this book, I will teach you the four components of the natural path to freedom from psoriasis that I followed instead of the conventional medical path. These components include diet, nutritional supplementation, detoxification, and meditation. You'll learn:

- Important medical definitions associated with psoriasis.
- The causes of autoimmunity—particularly the "chronic offenders."
- What to eat and not eat to halt symptoms of psoriasis and prevent them from returning.
- Ways to move your nervous system out of fight-or-flight mode.
- How to heal gut inflammation and restore your microbiome.
- The power of working with affirmations and how to rewire your brain to connect a healing mindset to a healing body.
- Which products in your home to eliminate (makeup, skin lotion, laundry detergent, and more) because

they contain ingredients your body cannot tolerate.

- A detailed ninety-day psoriasis-healing program which includes the renowned autoimmune protocol (AIP) diet, instructions for a five-day fasting-mimicking cleanse, lifestyle recipes for healing, and precise guidance with supplementation, detoxification, mindset, and nervous system restoration.

Who This Book Is For

This book is intended for those who no longer align with the medical treatments of drugs taken by mouth, drugs injected into the body, or drugs meant to be absorbed topically—meaning, through the skin. It is for those who are having difficulty getting past the contradictions of using chemicals to heal toxicity, inflammation, and systemic overwhelm.

This book is for those who feel inspired and are intrigued by the idea of addressing the root causes of psoriasis with a drug-free approach, thus shifting their paradigm of healing from outside-in to inside-out. It is a call to those who are willing to make their health a priority by spending time in the kitchen preparing healthful meals and exploring daily rituals and habits that can soothe the nervous system.

On the table is also the opportunity to examine their deeply ingrained beliefs regarding health and healing. The people who will find great value in this book are those who are willing to look at what may be uncomfortable truths about how the body becomes injured and how it heals, and how self-perpetuating harm may come from the negative manner in which we speak to ourselves.

If you've been told, like I was, that there is no cure for psoriasis, that it's a lifelong affliction that can go into remission (if you're lucky) but that, like a boogeyman, it lurks and waits to come back whenever it wants and with no warning. If you've been told that there are no predictable game changers available to you, and that beautiful skin is too lofty a dream for you, it's time to create a different truth for yourself.

Studies have shown that our bodies directly respond to the stories we tell ourselves. Thoughts we repeat persistently will be expressed symptomatically. For this reason alone, it's time to begin believing something different about what's possible for you and your body. So, if you are one of the 125 million people suffering from psoriasis, and despite anything you've been told to the contrary by your doctor, mother, brother, best friend, or preacher, smooth, radiant skin is most definitely possible for you.

The purpose of this book is to arm you with knowledge about true healing so that the pieces of you that are hidden in the shadows can surrender to the beauty that has always been there.

PART ONE

BACKGROUND

CHAPTER ONE

Medical Definitions

According to the National Psoriasis Foundation, psoriasis is an immune-mediated disease that causes inflammation in the body. An *immune-mediated disease* is any disease with an unclear cause that is characterized by inflammation and caused by a dysfunction in the immune system. With psoriasis, there may be visible signs of inflammation, such as raised plaques and scales on the skin. A plaque is a palpable, elevated skin lesion characterized by a flat surface and solid consistency. Plaques look different for people with different skin types and tones.[1]

Psoriasis occurs when an overactive immune system speeds up skin cell growth. Normal skin cells completely grow and shed (fall off) in a month. But in the case of psoriasis, the skin cells turn over in just three or four days, and instead of being shed, they pile up on the surface of the skin, causing plaques and flaking.[2]

Medical texts refer to psoriasis as being determined by excessive proliferation and impaired evolution of skin cells called *keratinocytes*. Keratinocytes represent the major cell type of the epidermis—the outermost of the seven layers of the skin—making up about 90 percent of the cells in it.[3]

Common symptoms of psoriasis include itching, burning, and stinging. Plaques and scales are commonly found on the elbows, knees, and scalp; and in more severe cases, they may also be found on the torso, face, and even the genitalia.[4]

Inflammation caused by psoriasis can impact other organs and tissues in the body. People with psoriasis may also experience other health conditions. One in three people with psoriasis, for example, will also develop psoriatic arthritis. Signs of this condition include swelling, stiffness, and pain in the joints and areas surrounding the joints. Psoriatic arthritis often goes undiagnosed, particularly in its milder forms.[5]

Symptoms of psoriasis often start between ages twelve and twenty-five, but they can start at any age. Men, women, and children of all ages can experience psoriasis.

Because psoriasis is autoimmune in nature, like all other autoimmune conditions it's referred to as *idiopathic,* meaning that its cause is unknown. The connotation of this word is unfortunate because it tends to reinforce the psoriasis sufferer's sense of powerlessness over the disease, frequently coupled with feelings of despair or hopelessness. But in fact, autoimmunity isn't without cause. It is associated with specific events, insults, and toxic exposures.

Most people who suffer from psoriasis become well-versed with the symptoms that define it and can rattle off a list of the various medical treatments they've tried.

I would like to propose the following definition for psoriasis, which will inform the practical measures we can take to heal psoriasis. Contrary to occurring for no reason, psoriasis is an autoimmune disorder whose expression comes about as a result of extreme stress being placed on both the nervous system and the digestive system—specifically on the microbiome in the gut. These factors result in inflammation and sloughing off of skin (our largest organ) as an attempt to detoxify the body.

Symptoms associated with psoriasis reflect the body's attempts to adapt to the injury caused by any number of possible emotional and environmental insults that we will explore in this book.

To repeat, *psoriasis is not random.* In general, its cause is known and documented repeatedly in the literature. Furthermore, psoriasis can be managed by decreasing inflammation, detoxifying the liver, healing an imbalanced gut, and perhaps, most importantly, by changing our mindset from hopeless victimization to grateful self-empowerment. I have found through my personal experience and deep conversations with other psoriasis sufferers that there tends to be a commonality to the way we think about ourselves and speak to ourselves when we wear an illness on the outside. When we change the damaging language and the resultant emotions, we often find the missing link to healing.

Gone are the days when psoriasis sufferers have to resolve themselves to spend over $20,000 per month on drugs with toxic side effects—a cost that seems only to create more stress and more disease.

Also gone are the days when we have to worry that we'll genetically pass on psoriasis to our kids and grandkids. This is the day that we interrupt the pattern.

The Traditional Approach to Psoriasis Treatment and the Health-Care Paradigm That Seeds It

The traditional approach that dermatologists and other medical doctors offer to treat psoriasis depends solely upon an array of powerful drugs that suppress the symptoms. Before we can discuss the problems with this treatment approach, I believe it's necessary to dissect the logic of the health-care paradigm that drives it, which is mainly interested in exercising control over natural intelligence and has little faith in the wisdom of the body.

How a society handles the treatment of any illness or health challenge depends on its beliefs about how the body gets sick, how the body stays healthy, and even what its shared definition of the term *health* is.

The concept of being *symptom-free* can be found at different locations along the spectrum from a state of disease to a state of health. We can be symptom free and very sick simultaneously. The most obvious example is with the presence of cancer before it becomes symptomatic or the instance of a major heart attack without a previous symptom. In these cases, people often will say things like "He was healthy until the day he died of that heart attack." Of course, this can't be true.

In our society's current health-care paradigm, we identify our symptoms, and then these symptoms, in and of themselves, become what we treat. We aim to reduce or eliminate symptoms, first and foremost, often without considering that the body may be attempting to express health through them. Take, for example, the direct correlation between childhood fevers and the meeting of developmental milestones or growth. In this case, not only is the fever benign but it's extremely beneficial to the child.

Another example of a symptom playing an important role in restoring the body to health is vomiting as a result of food poisoning. The body can save its own life (your life) by purging something potentially fatal.

Or take, for example, the raising of blood pressure in response to perceived danger in the environment as the body's attempt to help us mobilize to face it. The arousal state created by the fight-or-flight response is biologically intended to give us a chance to survive when we're being attacked; it's not meant to be our permanent state of being.

Our current health-care paradigm exhibits ambiguity about skin inflammation and rapid skin cell turnover being the body's attempt to rid itself of toxins and decrease systemic inflammation. However, it is my contention that this is exactly what the body is doing. As a chiropractor, my focus is primarily centered on restoring health to the nervous system. Due to the fact that psoriasis is autoimmune in nature and inflammation is an immune response known to be linked to stress, an optimally functioning spine and nervous system are absolutely necessary to return to a healing state.

In our society's current mainstream health-care paradigm, we're taught that most of our chronic illnesses, like heart disease and hypertension, type 1 diabetes, ADHD, depression and anxiety, *and* autoimmunity, are genetic in nature. This model also tells us that the body sometimes will simply begin to make functioning errors without an apparent cause. The mainstream treatments for any of these types of chronic conditions are brought in from the outside. I propose that we flip the plan and bring forth healing from the inside.

I believe that taking an outside-in approach to psoriasis treatment—meaning, taking pharmaceutical drugs like chemotherapy and biologics that have significant toxicity-linked side effects, or repeatedly using topical steroids in an attempt to create healing—is precisely where we've gone wrong. How could something known to cause chemical stress lead to healing?

This approach is a race we can never win. And I also believe it is why health outcomes continue to worsen for many people experiencing psoriasis symptoms, despite the increase in available medical interventions for this diagnosis. Instead, let's address the health of our gut microbiomes, clean up our nutrition, and remove harmful stressors to our nervous systems.

The conventional health-care model places us at the mercy of what our skin is doing, it denies us self-empowerment, and it does not offer us the tools we need to achieve true healing.

Like I said: The traditional approach to treating psoriasis is a masking strategy, at best.

CHAPTER TWO

Your Genes Are Not Your Destiny

The psychological stress and trauma attached to the lack of control I felt as I helplessly watched my skin erupt with redness and inflammation began in my teens and worsened in my twenties. I was respectively twenty-seven and thirty when I had my two beautiful boys with their perfectly unblemished, radiant-looking skin. Having been told for over a decade that psoriasis was genetic, when my sons were born my mind assaulted me with another layer of worry and fear. I was concerned that my children could wake up any day and suddenly find themselves plagued by terrible symptoms of psoriasis, like mine.

For many years, scientists in different countries have been investigating whether or not there are genes that make certain individuals more susceptible to developing psoriasis than others. They study whole families to see if they can find particular genetic markers.[1]

I think we need to be cautious in finger pointing the cause of autoimmunity of any kind to the genetic cards we've been dealt. If our genetic makeup is directly linked to the entire explanation for all the conditions a human being could potentially experience, how then do we explain the millions of cases of different diseases—cancer, heart disease, diabetes, and many other common chronic ailments among them—in which the inheritance of a particular genetic marker has never resulted in the manifestation of that particular illness? Surely this happens with individuals who carry the genetic markers for psoriasis, too.

We all know people, including ourselves, whose immediate families have a history of heart disease, diabetes, or cancer yet they never experience it themselves. Many of us never succumb to the illnesses that our grandparents, parents, and siblings share, despite our genetic similarities to them. There are even many studies showing that identical twins—people with exactly the same genetic profiles—will manifest a genetically linked illness completely differently. For these reasons and in order to move away from helplessness, I'd rather narrow my focus on the lifestyle choices and environmental factors which we know are linked to our condition and most importantly, on those which can directly lead to our healing.

The Human Genome Project

The Human Genome Project, which began in 1990 and ended in 2003, was an ambitious international effort to identify and decode all of the base gene pairs found within the human species.[2] The idea was that if we could decipher the chemical makeup of the entire human genome, then humanity might one day be able to eradicate all the chronic illnesses plaguing and killing us.

This project was sure to change everything, the researchers thought. They were hoping to help us biohack our way into optimal health.

The science was admittedly impressive, but the project came to an unexpectedly early end when the scientists involved made the surprising discovery that humans only have 20,000–25,000 genes as opposed to the 100,000 genes they expected to find.[3] In addition to the abrupt conclusion of the project, a fissure in the conversation of genetics as causality to chronic illness was born and scientists began seeing flaws in the theory that if we could identify the genetic culprits, we could build cures.

Suddenly, the Human Genome Project was no longer the beacon of hope for a "cured" future and no longer held the promise of saviorhood for our chronic illness epidemic. The whole story does continue to unravel and with the help of AI, the genetic connection to chronic illness may unravel a more thorough explanation but until then, we are in a holding pattern which leaves us no choice but to examine our lifestyle choices and environment.[4]

The Relatively New Science of Epigenetics

In January 2010, *Time* magazine reporter John Cloud wrote a widely circulated article entitled "Why Your DNA Isn't Your Destiny." It was around then that the world started exploring, or at least reporting on, the science of epigenetics.[5]

Much to the contrary of what we've been told and what we continue to be told by our doctors, preachers, sisters, and teachers, our genetic inheritance does not predict our health outcomes, nor does it explain how we uniquely express health and/or disease.

Epigenetics is the branch of science dating back to the 1950s that explores how our behaviors, our lifestyle choices, our habits, and our environments change the way our genes express themselves. In other words, what we know is that just because we may inherit a certain set of genes, whether or not those genes become expressed depends on the way we live our lives and to what we're exposed. As previously mentioned, identical twins, with identical genetic makeup at birth, can experience dramatically different health outcomes from one another depending on the environments they live and work in, and the kinds of choices they make.

In 2008, a group of epigeneticists proposed a definition of an epigenetic trait as a "stably heritable phenotype resulting from changes in a chromosome without alterations in the DNA sequence" to the attendees at a conference in Cold Spring Harbor, New York. This means that the gene doesn't change, but something in it does the equivalent of switching on or off, depending on conditions.[6]

Imagine that at birth, we're all given very similar LEGO® building sets with 25,000 pieces of different colors and shapes. The structures we individually build will be unique, with their differences largely based on our emotional, chemical, and physical environments and lifestyle choices. I might build a castle, and you might build a high-rise apartment building and someone else might build a mountain, all with similar sets of LEGO pieces.

The same is true for how we build our health outcomes.

The days of hopelessness and conversations are over that sound like "Well, my grandma had diabetes and my dad had diabetes; therefore, it's inevitable that I'll have diabetes, too."

We must now, with what we know, hold ourselves accountable for our health outcomes. This is not the same as assigning ourselves blame and guilt. What we're talking about is showing ourselves compassion when we feel unwell and gracefully taking responsibility for finding the solutions we need with the partnership of our healthcare team.

Having certainty over our how our health expresses itself can help us transform the feeling we have of being at the mercy of psoriasis (or another condition) into the feeling of capability. Then we can calmly focus on the bigger things in our lives while we navigate our way to improved, and ultimately optimal, wellness.

The sense of intentionally moving in the right direction requires us to take responsibility for our bodies. This means that we are making the choice to be active players with the power to change our outcomes. Taking responsibility shifts us from feeling like victims of our circumstances to being the captains of our health.

My sons are now men and they still have beautiful radiant skin and no autoimmune markers in their bloodstreams whatsoever. This good health, from an epigenetic perspective, isn't the result of luck or happenstance, but an expression of their genes as influenced by very deliberate, positive choices.

The chapters that follow will shed light on action steps you can take so that you can heal your psoriasis.

CHAPTER THREE

Commonly Prescribed Drugs

The average American adult is exposed to sixteen hours per year of direct-to-consumer pharmaceutical advertising on television alone. This doesn't include our exposure to pharmaceutical ads in magazines and newspapers, online, and on billboards in public places like arenas, stadiums, buses, and subways. And one sixth of these ads are for drugs for the treatment of psoriasis.[1]

To people who suffer with the skin-disfiguring symptoms of psoriasis, the inner contraction we feel when seeing such an ad can be palpable. Typically, the ads portray attractive actors chosen by casting directors because of their radiant, clear skin who probably have no idea what having psoriasis feels like. And as opposed to the artificially portrayed feelings of hope these ads are intended to impart, the viewer comes away feeling ashamed and inadequate.

Skyrizi, a psoriasis drug ranked #1 in 2025 as the most advertised drug in America, followed by Ozempic (GLP-1).[2] Despite there being over seventy different pharmaceutical drugs for psoriasis on the market today, psoriasis still plagues over 125 million people worldwide—3 percent of the human population—and it specifically affects over 7.5 million American adults.[3] Evidently, offering psoriasis treatment is an incredibly lucrative enterprise.

In 2025, pharmaceutical sales for the treatment of psoriasis generated 29.15 billion dollars in sales revenue. This annual revenue number is estimated to reach 72.99 billion dollars by 2034.[4] The pharmaceutical companies are predicting and wagering their financial resources on psoriasis becoming a bigger and bigger problem. They're counting on more diagnoses and more suffering. As an outside observer, it seems like actually curing psoriasis would be inconvenient and economically unbeneficial given the massive investments they've made.

According to the current mainstream medical model, treatment of psoriasis necessarily involves lifelong chemical interventions, rather than permanent healing or chemical intervention-free solutions.

But this begs the question: Why, if our psoriasis symptoms can only be "managed" with prescription medicines that we must take on a daily basis, are we then ever considered "better"? Are we then truly any healthier, or any more "healed," than we were before the introduction of those drugs?

Furthermore, are these drugs helping us or harming us?

I understand the desperation you might feel to have clear skin and less joint pain. Truly, I do. In pursuit of these goals, I allowed myself to be prescribed everything from steroids and methotrexate (a chemotherapy drug normally given to cancer patients). I even took a non-FDA-approved, mail-order steroid that could have killed a horse. I did this because I was willing to bear any side effect and future consequence if I could just get a respite from the painful emotions I felt when I looked at myself in the mirror—an action I avoided as much as possible.

Securing informed consent from a patient before they follow your advice seems to be a tricky proposition for doctors. It shouldn't be. Doctors should read us the literature line by line and discuss it comprehensively every time they prescribe a new drug for us. They should relay the side effects, research findings, and potential future ramifications for every drug, as well as the potential benefits, without exception. The decision to take any particular drug should be based on clarity and full disclosure.

But as we all know, this isn't the way the system works.

Here are some of the drugs I encountered before I discovered a natural way to heal.

Steroids

I was twelve when I was diagnosed with psoriasis. It started behind my ears, then appeared on my elbows, forearms, and knees. My mother, not knowing what else to do, took me to my family doctor, who prescribed me a topical corticosteroid. "Apply this cream, three time a day when needed. It should take care of it," he said.

Corticosteroids (topical steroids) are the most commonly prescribed treatment for psoriasis. In general, they work moderately well when applied regularly because they suppress inflammation. The catch is that this outcome is specific to usage. Unfortunately, flareups referred to as *rebound effects* can occur when their use is discontinued.[5] This often leads to a vicious cycle of symptoms and feeling like we need to apply more and more steroids.

With prolonged and more aggressive use, the common side effects of steroids (specific to the skin) can and will include thinning skin, spider veins, stretch marks, and skin breakouts.[6] The greatest risk of using them, however (one which is frequently omitted from dermatology websites and brochures on corticosteroid use) is the risk of adrenal suppression.

Prolonged use of topical steroids has been shown to cause damage to the adrenals glands similar to the damage of systemic oral steroid use. Retrospective studies of psoriasis sufferers with skin lesions on 10 percent or more of their bodies who made chronic use of topical steroids showed a significant increase in "silent" adrenal insufficiency—meaning, the condition remains hidden until triggered by a trauma or stress to the body where the pendulum can swing very rapidly into adrenal crisis.[7]

The adrenal glands are located above the kidneys. These glands produce hormones that help regulate the metabolism, immune system, and blood pressure. They also produce hormones that help us respond and adapt to stress.

Adrenal suppression can cause significant fatigue, low blood pressure, body aches, lightheadedness, hair loss, and skin discoloration.[8] Importantly, when the adrenal glands are damaged, this affects how well we adapt to our environment in response to stressors. If our ability is diminished, it can rapidly lead to more serious illness and perpetuate an autoimmune cascade. The most common secondary symptom of adrenal failure is the development of thyroid disease, which is a significantly growing health problem in today's society.[9]

Calcitriol: The Active Form of Vitamin D

When I was fifteen, my parents and I moved to Florida, where I lived for three years. I subjected myself to regular sunburn because the combination of sun and steroid was so successful at keeping my psoriasis symptoms at bay that sun damage was the least of my worries.

By the time I was pursuing undergraduate studies, back in my hometown of Ottawa, Canada, with its long winters, my weekly sunburns were no longer available and my symptoms got worse. Despite heavy corticosteroid use, I now had psoriasis on my face, and specifically, the redness around my eyebrows and my ears was very severe. It was in Ottawa that I saw a dermatologist for the second time. He prescribed what he referred to as a "simple vitamin D cream" to use along with the corticosteroid cream.

Calcitriol is the only vitamin D3 ointment available to consumers in the United States, and in my opinion, which is based on reading numerous research studies, it appears to be the safest topical option.[10]

Topical vitamin D3 can be effective because it acts mainly on the vitamin D receptors in skin cells to regulate and slow down their growth. Vitamin D3 also inhibits inflammatory processes much like a steroid but in my opinion, in a safer manner.

At the age of twenty-two, I started chiropractic graduate school in Upstate New York. Being from Canada, in order to receive a student visa to matriculate in the United States, I was required to show proof of childhood vaccinations. But when I was five, our house had burned to the ground, and all my early childhood vaccine records were lost.

Back then, in the era prior to electronic health records, vaccine records were kept on a paper card that you filed in your medical dossier in a filing cabinet. Having lost this card, I couldn't prove that I'd received the required vaccines. The only solution (I was told) was to vaccinate me for all the vaccines that I'd already received, and then some. This was done in one sitting and without me giving *properly informed* consent. I consented, but I really didn't know enough to question what the doctor was doing—and after all, I needed to acquiesce to this requirement in order to attend the graduate school of my choice.

Within four months of receiving the mandated vaccines, the psoriasis plaques on my body had more than tripled in size and location.

Psoriasis as a documented side effect of vaccination will be discussed further on.

Three and a half years later, my graduate school sweetheart, Darin, and I were engaged to be married and preparing for life in the United States after school. As part of the permanent residency application process, we had to present ourselves for an interview and physical examination. I can't honestly remember the details, but I do recall that in order to receive my "green card," I was subjected, once again, to another full round of vaccinations. Again, nobody informed me of the potential side effects I could experience.

Within six weeks, my body was covered with severe plaques once more.

I was desperate. My parents, in a loving attempt to help me—being that my fiancé and I were still broke chiropractic students—created an opportunity for me to go to one of the most renowned dermatology clinics in New York City. I waited anxiously for over a month for the appointment, counting the minutes until a doctor, any doctor, would help me get by life back. I eagerly walked into the clinic with the thousand dollars required just to walk in the door. The clinic looked like a five-star hotel and everybody working at the front desk looked like they modeled in their spare time. I was relieved to be in a place that promised to return me to myself.

Darin stayed in the waiting room of the dermatology clinic while I waited for the doctor in the examination room. I sat on a cold, metal exam table, wearing a short, practically sleeveless, thin cotton gown that opened at the back. The nicely coiffed doctor walked in with his white coat and bright white teeth and quickly glanced at my chart. He asked me to take a look at my back first, then looked at my arms and legs and finally at my abdomen. I'm not sure if he couldn't bring himself to look at my lesioned skin or if he just didn't want to look, but his apparent antipathy for my condition was palpable. All I could do was sit there, holding my breath, feeling frozen in time.

Twenty-two years later, I don't think I've ever felt more alone than I felt in that room with that doctor. I still fail to understand how somebody with his training and credentials could make anybody feel so small, so invisible, and so judged in such a short period of time. If I could have melted into the floor and disappeared, I would have.

As I sat there reluctantly showing the doctor my skin, which he was trying not to look at, he told me that this would never resolve on its own and that yes, I would probably be like this forever. He then proceeded to tell me that with the severity of "coverage," topicals were no longer appropriate. In his opinion, the only option for me was the chemotherapy drug methotrexate. This is marketed under various brand names, including Jylamvo, Rheumatrex, Trexall, and Xatmep.

Methotrexate

Methotrexate is said to sometimes be effective because it binds to the skin enzymes responsible for rapid cell turnover, thereby slowing down the replication of skin cells.

The dermatologist who prescribed it for me did proceed to secure some of the informed consent associated with methotrexate for somebody of my age and gender, which included possible effects on fertility. He failed to inform me, though, that methotrexate also could cause liver damage and would increase my risk of lymphoma, bone marrow toxicity, and infection (due to reducing my white blood cell count).[11]

I took the prescription—and what was left of my pride—and made my way up front to pay the supermodels at the reception desk. As I walked out to meet my fiancé in the waiting room, I could see the hope and love in his eyes. It wasn't until we were in the elevator and headed down to our car that I began sobbing.

Out of helplessness, I decided to start taking the methotrexate because it seemed like my only hope. The drug came in pill form and I was advised not to touch it with my hands when taking it. This was confusing advice, considering I would be swallowing it. I was warned that my hair could fall out, my fertility could be affected, and I could feel tired, sluggish, and sick. None of it mattered because the only thing I had on my mind was the grand prize of healing my skin.

After taking the pills for three to four weeks, my skin actually got much worse, so I stopped taking it. It turns out that this is a known potential consequence of methotrexate treatment. Today, twenty-five years later, I'm grateful for that moment because I know that my body was taking the best care of me possible by making it clear that consuming such a toxic drug was not what would heal me.

If the drugs we take create toxicity, and if we have to sign waivers and get regular blood tests to make sure our organs aren't failing while we're on them, even if our skin gets better, and even if we become completely symptom-free, is there a chance that we're getting sicker? Or maybe even *much* sicker?

And is this acceptable?

Biologics: Monoclonal Antibodies, Vaccines, Hormones, and Other Drugs

My journey toward real healing with psoriasis truly began as the biologics known as *monoclonal antibodies* were just beginning to emerge. Some were tried and abandoned. Hundreds were approved. Because of good timing, I was spared the difficult decision of taking them, which back then, not knowing what I know now, I surely would have. I'm grateful I figured out a different, natural solution for healing my psoriasis.

Biologics like Enbrel, Humira, Skyrizi, and Remicade are said only to target specific parts of the immune system. Essentially, they are cloned proteins that bind to a single type of receptor in cells. Biologics used to treat psoriasis and psoriatic arthritis block the action of a specific type of immune cell called a *T-cell.* They can also block the effect of signaling proteins in the immune system that are responsible for the inflammatory response, both tumor necrosis factor and various interleukins. These drugs may alleviate the symptoms of psoriasis, but they do not cure it. Furthermore, they must often be taken for life or else the psoriasis returns.[12]

A prominent study published in *The Journal of Allergy and Clinical Immunology* states that "another autoimmune consequence of biologic therapy is the induction of skin psoriasis."[13] In this paper, the authors discuss the finding that many of those taking biologics for conditions like rheumatoid arthritis, IBS, and ankylosing spondylitis frequently develop psoriasis as well. They reference other studies and the products' own package inserts stating that biologic therapy can have the unintended consequence of altering the immune system overall, thus perpetuating autoimmunity.

Other potential side effects of biologics include severe infections potentially causing death, allergic reactions, nervous system problems like vision problems, tingling, and weakness, blood problems, heart failure, and liver problems, lymphoma and other cancers, strokes, and various autoimmune diseases.[14]

Patients on biologic drugs should have blood work done every three to twelve months to rule out pathology, severe infection, and tuberculosis.[15]

Agreeing to receive this type of invasive therapy seems to me like playing Russian roulette. That being said, I also understand and sympathize with what it's like to be desperate and just to want the problem to be handled, at least for a while.

Other documented side effects of biologic drugs include full-body rashes after injection (including the development of lupus-like syndrome), shortness of breath, cardiac reactions (including heart failure), severe infections, reactivation of hepatitis B, and central nervous system reactions.[16]

Coal Tar Products

After I had my first son, at the age of twenty-eight, the hormonal changes of pregnancy, giving birth, and breastfeeding, along with the exhaustion and depletion that came with caring for this love of my life, my first born, caused my skin to flare tremendously.

Because I was nursing and couldn't take or use steroids, the dermatologist I was seeing at the time gave me a white plastic jar of coal tar that I would spread all over my body before bed at night three or four times a week. I distinctly remember the smell of that tar, as I'm sure my husband and possibly my son do as well. I would cover myself up with it before bed and then proceed to wear cotton pajamas over it so that I wouldn't stain the bed sheets. The pajamas would stick to the tar and my fingernails would blacken from all the scratching at the incessant itchiness caused by the tar, which had a drying effect.

The mornings after I used the tar, I would go to the dermatologist's office to stand naked in a UVB booth for ten to fifteen minutes. This routine wasn't conducive to the already lacking "sexy time" that comes with having a baby. I'm sure my husband loved all of this . . . said no one ever.

Coal tar has been used for over a hundred years for the treatment of psoriasis. The National Psoriasis Foundation suggests trying coal tar if the psoriasis is present on less than 3 percent of the skin. Aside from the extreme tediousness of using coal tar, research has demonstrated an increased risk of cancer from combining the use of coal tar with UVB exposure.[17]

I suppose the proverbial elephant in the room in the discussion of psoriasis treatment is the fact that all the typical treatments, all the lotions and potions and pills and injections, come with the risk of significant side effects, one of which is the risk of worsening the psoriasis symptoms. It's difficult to understand why, at this point, considering there are 125 million psoriasis sufferers worldwide and the medical industry has thrown so many millions of dollars at the problem, there isn't yet a reliable natural protocol that can be recommended to people with psoriasis as the first and least invasive approach they should try.

None of the drugs and medical treatments I tried over the years worked as hoped. Some made me sick, and some made my skin worse. It wasn't until I changed the way I was approaching my symptoms that I actually healed. That's when my entire life changed.

CHAPTER FOUR

Four Key Causes of Autoimmunity

Medical literature states that, in most cases, psoriasis begins in adulthood, but for me and many of the people I've had the privilege of helping heal autoimmunity, the onset of psoriasis occurred during the teen years.

If by now we can agree, or at least entertain the notions, that psoriasis isn't necessarily a genetic hand-me-down and that it doesn't simply appear out of nowhere, for no reason, then we are ready to explore the known causes of autoimmunity.

As we've discussed, illness doesn't happen to us without reason. The body harbors more innate intelligence than this. Healthy bodies don't just randomly become chronically weakened and sick. Diseases, including autoimmune diseases, always are the result of one or several causative factors.

If this is true, then it begs the question: *What is the cause of illness?*

There are four key causes of illness. These four causes are related to each and every illness in existence. No matter how much we want to complicate and fancify our health problems, they always originate from some combination of physical stress (including exposure to electromagnetic fields), chemical stress (including exposure to toxins and allergens), genetic influences, and emotional stress.

It would be foolish to assume (or hope) we could avoid being exposed to stress of any kind. We all know that avoidance of stress altogether is impossible. Fortunately, our bodies are built to handle most of the stressors we encounter. Autoimmune problems arise either when our level of stress becomes too great for us to adapt to it all at once, or when our adaptation capabilities have been reduced to the point where even the most innocuous stressor causes the pendulum of health to swing in the direction of degeneration and disease.

Key Cause 1: Physical Stress

Studies have shown that physical injuries, particularly traumatic injuries such as falls, car accidents, and sports injuries, can be the trigger for an autoimmune state to develop. Some injuries happen more gradually, over time, in the form of repetitive actions like sitting forty hours a week at a desk in front of a computer and holding a mouse, or while driving a truck or a taxicab for a living. Postural complaints and mechanical injuries frequently arise from the stress of these types of work and lifestyle habits.

There are studies indicating that concussion injuries can lead to the development of autoimmune diseases. Studies performed on both soldiers and athletes have demonstrated that traumatic brain injuries can trigger inflammation and immune regulatory factors involved with autoimmune disease.[1]

My psoriasis initially manifested itself shortly after an accident in which I fell down a twenty-five-foot ravine onto a bed of large rocks while driving a three-wheeler ATV. I hit my head and lost consciousness for an unknown period of time. When I came to, I was nearly a mile away from the site of the crash, on foot and dazedly walking through a field with no recollection as to how I'd gotten there. I had severe contusions on my torso and egg-sized masses all over my head.

At the time, my family's approach (offered to me with all the love in their hearts) was simply to put me in a warm bath with a glass of milk. Back then, with French Canadians, this was the approach for most accidents, including near-death experiences. I didn't go to the doctor.

Sudden injuries and repetitive stress injuries affect the function of the nervous system. If the nervous system is the master controller for all organs and functions in the body as well as serving as the foundation for health and healing, anything that shocks the nervous system has the potential to impede health. Sudden injuries and repetitive physical stress invariably affect overall functioning of the body. The question is: *How well can the body adapt to it?*

Once the nervous system's ability to communicate with all the vital organs, tissues, and systems is interfered with, our healing mechanisms are dampened. My professional expertise as a chiropractor lies in helping my patients' bodies restore and maintain proper function.

Because the nervous system is largely housed in the spine, corrective and lifestyle-driven chiropractic care is essential to ensure a full return to nervous system flow and function. Chiropractic care helps the brain and nervous system heal, and in my experience, regular chiropractic care is an absolutely essential part of the healing journey for people with autoimmunity.

In addition to injuries, electromagnetic field (EMF) exposure is a physical stressor that people with psoriasis ought to avoid. Exposure to EMFs in the form of prolonged use of cellular devices, 5G and 6G (soon to come at the time of this writing), and continued close proximity to routers and wireless devices has been increasing for decades. In 2004, the World Health Organization held a special meeting in Prague to discuss the specifics as to the ramifications of EMFs. It was at this meeting that five precursors to disease were identified: physical trauma to the central nervous system, exposure to chemical toxins in the environment, exposure to biological stressors like bacteria, viruses and parasites, and depleted immune and nervous system function. Most important for our purposes here, what they found was that there is also evidence that "exposure to electromagnetic fields can amplify immune system dysfunction, including immune suppression, autoimmunity and hyperinflammation."[2]

Key Cause 2: Chemical Stress

In my personal case, soon after my ATV accident, there were two definite and specific encounters with chemical toxins—in the form of medication—that immediately and undeniably triggered a storm of psoriasis. My healing journey later on required the acknowledgment and awareness of the immense load these toxins put on my body, which for me originally tipped the scales of my health toward inflammation and autoimmunity. My system was doing its best to detoxify by expressing the symptoms of psoriasis in the manner it did, but it was uncomfortable.

Before we discuss different kinds of toxins and the management of chemical stress, it should be noted that I was shocked and dismayed, as I unraveled the truth of the sources of my own toxicity, at the lack of information I was provided before encouraging me to take powerful pharmaceutical medications. Informed consent procedures should have been followed by my health-care providers prior to introducing these drugs—with their very specific known risks and side effects.

As a layperson, I didn't know the risks or side effects. I simply trusted that my "health leaders" would hold themselves accountable and inform me of anything to which I might have a reaction or which could deleteriously affect my health. They didn't.

Before we put the uncertainty of the past behind us and look to the future, let's identify and discuss the toxins known to be linked with psoriasis. If you are being exposed to such toxins currently, I recommend that you promptly eliminate them from your environment and lifestyle. If your toxic exposure occurred in the past, even if you are no longer being exposed to any of these substances, I will teach you how to rid your body of them through detoxification in order for functional healing to occur.

Here we go.

Antibiotics

Antibiotics are a known trigger of psoriasis flareups. According to reports from people with psoriasis that I've read or heard, medical doctors will frequently deny the link and dismiss their patients' concerns about antibiotics. This being said, the link is prevalent in the peer-reviewed medical literature and any unfounded invalidation does not discount the need for a careful approach.[3]

Ninety years ago, antibiotics were hailed as miracle drugs. Antibiotics are indeed frequent life savers and their effectiveness is scientifically sound. The overuse of antibiotics, however, is prevalent, with many people having been prescribed dozens of courses of antibiotics by the age of eighteen. Ideally, over the course of a lifetime, a person should not require the need for antibiotics more than once or twice at the very most; but for many, this quota is met in toddlerhood.

A growing number of studies have shown that taking a single course of antibiotics, even short term, can alter the makeup of the bacterial species living in the gut. Recent studies have shown that antibiotics alter the health and diverse makeup of this microbiome. Studies also demonstrate that this dysbiosis can occur after a single course of antibiotics and that the deleterious change can persist for months to several years.[4]

Because psoriasis (as well as all other autoimmune disease) is directly related to damage in the gut lining, damage to the beneficial bacteria in the intestinal lining can be detrimental. One of the ways that antibiotics will specifically alter the diversity and balance of the gut microbiome is by altering the microbial metabolites of the gut that are involved with the fermentation of undigested dietary fiber. Metabolites are particles produced by the trillions of microbes in the gut which play a vital role with the balance of our overall health. This altered metabolite state is directly connected to inflammation, particularly inflammation of the epithelial cells lining the gut, which also are among the most abundant cells covering the skin.[5]

Although all antibiotics should be used with caution and be combined with proper gut-healing protocols (see

Chapter 7), the medical literature points toward tetracycline, in particular, as being very specifically problematic for the worsening of psoriasis symptoms.[6]

In the event that an antibiotic should become necessary to overcome an infection, a high-quality probiotic should be taken simultaneously, along with the ingestion of microbiome-diversifying foods.

Cadmium: A Metal

A study published in 2017 demonstrates the link between the likelihood of having psoriasis and elevated levels of blood cadmium.[7] Cadmium is a toxic metal found in some foods, including cereals and cereal products, rice, starchy vegetables, and tobacco. It is also found in old batteries.

The body has a difficult time detoxifying itself from cadmium, and the half-life of cadmium in the human body is ten years.

The most highly concentrated form of readily present cadmium people tend to be exposed to appears to be through cigarette smoke, including when inhaled through second-hand smoke. Cigarette smoking has been linked with a higher prevalence of psoriasis.[8] There is increasing evidence of metal toxicity in our society due to the presence of cadmium in the liquids and aerosols that come with vaping and e-cigarettes. These metal toxicity levels have been measured in the blood, urine, plasma, and saliva of e-cigarette users.[9]

All smokers (and I used to be one of them) are aware that they should quit. No smoker ever said that they didn't know smoking was harmful—and continually being told what you already know is excessively irritating. As it relates to psoriasis, please do know, however, that if you are a smoker, quitting smoking and then detoxifying your body of cadmium could be the starting point for permanently healing your psoriasis.

Specifically, elevated blood cadmium interferes with the body's assimilation of zinc, an essential mineral that aids in the healing of psoriasis. Zinc supplementation is therefore necessary for those with psoriasis, particularly for those who smoke still or formerly smoked.

Anti-Malarial Drugs

Exacerbation and induction of psoriasis with the use of the malarial drugs chloroquine and hydroxychloroquine, the two most commonly prescribed oral anti-malaria medications, are well documented and widely acknowledged in the literature.[10] This is thought to be directly connected to the inhibition of an enzyme (transglutaminase) in the skin which has influence over skin proliferation.

In 2017, my husband and I took our eight- and ten-year-old boys to travel and live in our Volkswagen Eurovan through Colombia, Ecuador, and Peru for five months. It was an adventure like no other, and we had big decisions to make regarding precautionary measures. Antimalarial drugs (taken preventatively) were highly recommended by the pharmacist and even by our family naturopath. Upon informing myself of the side effects, including the documented risk of depression and mental health trauma, as well as the risk of the exacerbation of psoriasis, we decided to become well-informed as to the symptoms of malaria instead.

We took the antimalarial drugs with us and our plan (as discusses with our pharmacist) was to take the drugs as needed if we ever began experiencing the symptoms of malarial infection. We never had a problem I am glad to report.

NSAIDS

Taking nonsteroidal anti-inflammatory drugs (NSAIDS) for pain management, particularly when they're being used regularly both systemically (orally) and topically, is known to worsen psoriasis symptoms.[11] These drugs are often taken for inflammatory arthritis and therefore are often used by people suffering from psoriatic arthritis. This creates the risk of a vicious cycle where we're taking a drug to handle the inflammatory symptoms of psoriatic arthritis while the very drug we're taking exacerbates our psoriasis symptoms.

Examples of NSAIDs are aspirin, ibuprofen (Advil), naproxen (Aleve), celecoxib (Celebrex), diclofenac

(Voltaren), fenoprofen (Nalfon), indomethacin (Indocin), and ketorolac (Toradol).

A natural alternative to NSAIDS would be an oral dose of homeopathic *Arnica montana,* which, for some people, acts as a powerful painkiller.

The daily implementation of turmeric supplementation is also a very effective natural remedy for reducing overall inflammation; it can help relieve both the pain and the inflammation related to psoriasis.

Beta Blockers

Beta blockers are most prevalent in the treatment of cardiovascular diseases, like hypertension, ischemic heart disease, arrhythmia, and congestive heart failure. But they are also used to treat non-cardiovascular diseases, like hyperthyroidism, glaucoma, migraine, and anxiety. They are effective at relaxing the smooth tissue in the heart and blood vessels because they block epinephrine and norepinephrine.

In 2022, an astounding 30 million Americans were using beta blockers, so it was perhaps inevitable that some were people experiencing psoriasis. Research now does indicate that beta blockers are known to both trigger the onset of and to exacerbate the symptoms of psoriasis.[12] It is believed that this occurs due to interference with inflammatory mediators.

Examples of beta-blocking drugs include Atenolol, Betaxolol, Bisoprolol, Esmolol, Metoprolol, and Nebivolol.

Lithium: A Metal

Lithium has been used since the 1970s for the treatment of mental-health disorders, particularly the manic episodes of bipolar disorders. Brands of lithium include Eskalith, Eskalith-CR, and Lithobid.

Consumption of lithium has been connected to the exacerbation of preexisting psoriasis as well as to the onset of novel psoriasis. Psoriasis flareups occur in 50 percent of those taking it. This side effect is largely due to its effect on the liver.

A 2017 review in *The Journal of Psoriasis and Psoriatic Arthritis* states that taking supplements of the sugar inositol, which is naturally found in some fruits, beans, and grains, helps to reduce liver congestion. In this way, it can help mitigate lithium-induced symptoms of psoriasis.[13]

ACE Inhibitors

ACE inhibitors, or *angiotensin converting enzymes* inhibitors, which are commonly prescribed for high blood pressure, heart failure, and chronic kidney disease, have been shown repeatedly and through meta-analyses of groups of studies to significantly induce the onset of psoriasis and exacerbate existing psoriasis symptoms. It has been shown that ACE inhibitors behave as a trigger for psoriasis because they increase the infiltration of inflammatory cells into tissues, thereby proliferating the spread and severity of skin plaques.[14]

Interferons

Interferons are drugs used to treat hepatitis B and C, lymphoma, leukemia, malignant melanoma, multiple sclerosis, and genital warts. It is well documented that interferons alpha, beta, and gamma have a strong association with the onset of as well as the exacerbation of psoriasis. Due to this well-established risk, medical guidelines advised against the use of interferons as a treatment for persons with a psoriasis diagnosis.[15]

Biologics

A biologic is any drug made from a living organism. The ones that are most likely to trigger psoriasis flareups are monoclonal antibodies and vaccines. Although some kinds of biologics are prescribed to treat psoriasis, one of their side effects is the documented worsening of the condition of psoriasis if you stop taking them. This troubling contradiction creates boundless confusion among patients, as do the side effects of many other pharmaceutical treatments given for psoriasis. If you are already taking monoclonal antibodies or considering taking them, please reread the information on biologics that I supplied in Chapter 3.

NOTE: Always consult with your medical provider as to the best approach when discontinuing the use of the drugs or making changes to any of the medications discussed above.

Childhood Vaccinations

The vaccination–autoimmune condition link is one I have been passionately discussing and studying for nearly three decades.

Prior to 1986, American children received three vaccines for seven illnesses. Two of these were combination injections for diphtheria-tetanus-pertussis and for measles-mumps-rubella. They also got a single polio vaccine. Thus totaling twenty-four doses by age eighteen. Due to the large amounts of money spent in the courts with vaccine injury claims, in 1986, through the Childhood National Vaccine Injury Act, the American government indemnified the pharmaceutical companies and began protecting them from liability for vaccine-specific injuries. To this day, if a person experiences a vaccine injury, the pharmaceutical maker of said vaccine is protected against all legal repercussions. They cannot be sued.

The act states: "No vaccine manufacturer shall be liable in a civil action for damages arising from a vaccine-related injury or death."[16]

The Vaccine Injury Compensation Program created by the U.S. Health Resources and Services Administration in conjunction with the 1986 Childhood National Vaccine Injury Act is in place to provide a federal no-fault system for compensating people for vaccine-related injuries or death by establishing a claim procedure involving the U.S. Court of Federal Claims and Office of Special Masters.[17] Despite this act, compensation and acknowledgment of vaccine injuries are nearly impossible to obtain. The process is littered with red tape, making it tedious, expensive, and exhausting to pursue a claim.

Fast forward. Today, in the 2020s, a child whose family is adhering to the mandated childhood vaccine schedule receives sixty-nine doses in total of an assortment of sixteen vaccines by age eighteen. The pharmaceutical companies continue to be free of liability for injuries.

Liability immunity also applies to adult vaccinations such as the vaccines for pneumonia, shingles, and Covid-19.

Here's the trouble with vaccines. In 1985, less than 10 percent of children had a chronic health condition. In 2025, More than 40 percent of children currently have a chronic health condition.[18] In some cases, instead of making our immune systems stronger, vaccines may be damaging them.

Vaccine-associated autoimmune disorders are well documented, and specifically, there is a known vaccine connection to both the onset and the exacerbation of psoriasis.[19] Aside from the numerous anecdotal reports of psoriasis being triggered by vaccination, the vaccine–psoriasis link is well documented scientifically and warnings of psoriasis as a side effect to vaccination are included in many vaccine product package inserts.

According to research, vaccination can trigger and exacerbate psoriasis symptoms. Several specific studies and/or package inserts document an association between the specific vaccines discussed below and the onset of psoriasis and/or the exacerbation of psoriasis.

Let's look at a few of them together.

The Adenovirus Vaccine. The package insert for the adenovirus vaccine states:

> *The safety and effectiveness of Adenovirus Type 4 and Type 7 Vaccine, Live, Oral in immunocompromised individuals has not been evaluated.*

It also states that those receiving immunosuppressive therapy (like biologics) should avoid exposure to anyone having been vaccinated for adenovirus for twenty-eight days following vaccination due to shedding. Furthermore:

> *There are no data regarding the use of Adenovirus Vaccine, Live, Oral concomitantly with immunosuppressive therapies (like corticosteroids and biologics).*[20]

The Diphtheria, Pertussis, and Tetanus Vaccine (DPT). The DPT vaccine package insert for Infanrix states that a commonly reported side effect includes "Skin and Subcutaneous Tissue Disorders."[21]

The DPT vaccine package insert for Daptacel, a comparable vaccine, states side effects of immune system disorders, including "Hypersensitivity, allergic reaction, anaphylactic reaction, edema, face edema, swelling face, pruritus, rash generalized and other types of skin rashes including those which are erythematous, macular, maculopapular."[22]

The Smallpox Vaccine. The U.S. Centers for Disease Control (CDC) Smallpox vaccination fact sheet states the following.

> *Persons who have ever been diagnosed with eczema or atopic dermatitis should not be vaccinated, even if the condition is not currently active. These patients are at high risk of developing eczema vaccinatum, a potentially severe and sometimes fatal complication."*

Additionally, the insert states:

> *Persons with household contacts that have a history of eczema or atopic dermatitis, irrespective of disease severity or activity, should not be vaccinated.*
>
> *If the potential vaccinee or any of their household contacts have other acute, chronic, or exfoliative skin conditions (e.g., burns, impetigo, chicken pox, contact dermatitis, shingles, herpes, severe acne, severe diaper dermatitis with extensive areas of denuded skin, or psoriasis), they are at risk for inadvertent autoinoculation of the affected skin with vaccinia virus and should not be vaccinated until the condition(s) resolves.*[23]

The Departments of Health in several different states include people with psoriasis in the category of those who shouldn't be vaccinated for smallpox.[24]

Covid-19 Vaccines. Although so much more recent, the Covid-19 vaccine has countless and numerous literature reports of triggering psoriasis. A comprehensive review of the literature pertaining to the various Covid-19 vaccines and their association with psoriasis was done in 2022. The findings included seven studies reporting new onset of psoriasis following vaccination, thirty-two studies reporting flares and exacerbations, and four studies reporting both.[25]

The exacerbation of existing psoriasis or an occurrence of new-onset psoriasis has been linked to all Covid-19 vaccines, including the mRNA vaccines developed by Moderna and BioNTech/Pfizer. Psoriasis onset was reported following first, second, and third vaccine doses; however studies show that psoriasis flares are mostly linked to the second dose. The onset of psoriasis as a new development typically occurred between two and twenty-one days after administration of the vaccine, and the onset of flareups for individuals with preexisting psoriasis occurred anytime between one and ninety days after vaccination.[26]

The HPV Vaccine. In 2014, Gardasil, which is given to both young girls and boys (ages nine to twenty-six), was introduced to protect against human papilloma virus (HPV), which in some cases is connected to cervical cancer. The vaccine package insert documents a "Summary of Girls and Women 9 Through 26

Years of Age Who Reported an Incident Condition Potentially Indicative of a Systemic Autoimmune Disorder After Enrollment in Clinical Trials of GARDASIL including the condition of Psoriasis."[27]

It also should be noted that the insert mentions many other potential autoimmune symptoms arising following Gardasil vaccination, including, but not limited to, autoimmune thyroiditis, lupus, rheumatoid arthritis, celiac disease, and type-2 diabetes.[28]

The Measles, Mumps, and Rubella (MMR) Vaccine. The package vaccine insert for MMR states: "*Do not administer M-M-R II vaccine to individuals who are immunodeficient or immunosuppressed due to disease or medical therapy*" —meaning, a person with autoimmunity and/or a person who is taking a biologic drug should not receive the vaccine.

The insert also states that the MMR vaccine should not be administered to an individual with a family history or congenital or hereditary immunodeficiency.[29]

Additionally, there are reports in the literature of exacerbations and onset of psoriasis occurring following receipt of an influenza vaccine, a tuberculosis vaccine, or a pneumococcal polysaccharide vaccine.[30]

Overall, it stands to reason that if someone's immune system is under stress due to an autoimmune disease such as psoriasis, there should be caution with the introduction of drugs meant to trigger and modulate the immune system artificially, such as traditional live or attenuated vaccinations, as well as the newer mRNA vaccines.

How to Ensure That Your Doctor Gives You the Information You Need Before Treatment

Before you agree to receive a vaccination or take medication, it is perfectly reasonable to ask many questions about documented risks and side effects. Every pharmaceutical product comes with a product insert document which can be requested in person and/or found online at the FDA Online Labels Repository (https://labels.fda.gov) by proprietary name. All package inserts include contraindications, warnings, and precautions, and lists of adverse reactions, drug interactions, and clinical studies.

Informed consent procedures are often lacking or nonexistent when we're being presented with the very serious choice of vaccination. A thorough informed consent procedure should acknowledge and bring the potential recipient's awareness to the risks of developing autoimmunity that arise from being injected not only with live or attenuated viruses, but also with the ingredients they are blended with, like aluminum, ethylene glycol, formaldehyde, egg whites, and sodium chloride.

A thorough assessment of a person's immune system, including their historical use of immunosuppressive drugs such as corticosteroids and biologics, as well as a thorough family history to identify any familial risk of autoimmunity should be conducted prior to giving someone the MMR vaccine. Unfortunately, as many of us have experienced, these protocols are assumed to be followed, but rarely are in reality. Taking steps to ensure your health-care provider is aware that you have an autoimmune condition or a family history of autoimmunity, as well as any history of having taken immune-suppressive drugs like steroids or biologics, will help protect you against drug interactions and immune system damage.

Key Cause 3: Genetic Predispositions

After my boys were born, Darin and I realized that if we protected our children from exposure to certain toxins and taught them to lead healthful lifestyles, then we had the power to interrupt the generational pattern of psoriasis in our family. And we did.

The science of epigenetics has revealed that even if we inherit a specific gene predisposing us to develop a health condition like heart disease, cancer, or high cholesterol, the illness will only manifest if we are exposed to environmental conditions that our bodies' deem toxic and which overload their capacities to handle. Our lifestyle choices and personal experiences are significant factors preserving or damaging our health. This explains why out of five women in a family that has a history of breast cancer, for example, only one or two may develop cancer while the others go through their lives unscathed.

In the case of psoriasis, the fact that a person inherits a gene associated with autoimmunity increases their likelihood of developing autoimmunity, but the expression of this gene's potential does not occur unless the person is exposed to an environmental trigger of some kind. In the case of autoimmunity, as we have been discussing, there is usually a combination of triggers. Each of us has to do our own sleuthing to uncover the origins of our own psoriasis.

Methylenetetrahydrofolate reductase (MTHFR) is the enzyme responsible for breaking down the amino acid homocysteine. High homocysteine levels can lead to a host of diseases.[31] MTHFR is also a key regulatory enzyme for the activation of B vitamins, especially the metabolism of folate. Essentially, those with MTHFR gene mutation have trouble converting folate from the food they eat into methylfolate (L-5-MTHF), the bioavailable folate enzyme needed for the synthesis of DNA and methylation. In simpler terms, a MTHFR gene mutation interferes with the body's ability to properly methylate.[32] Methylation dynamically regulates our physiological responses to changes in the external environment, like getting a vaccination.

It is estimated that over 50 percent of the world's population has a MTHFR gene mutation of some kind. It is rarer that people inherit the same mutation from both parents. A specific variation of this gene known as C677T is commonly found in those suffering with autoimmunity and psoriasis—and there is a test you can take for this.[33]

Methylation is a biochemical process that is ongoing in every cell in our bodies starting from the time we are zygotes. It influences genetic expression, cellular repair, and neurotransmitter balance.[34] Psoriatic skin lesions appear to be associated with changes in DNA methylation.[35]

Because so many people have MTHFR gene mutations, it is essential that each of us discuss our risk of autoimmune damage and psoriasis with our doctors. This is how a person with a gene mutation will know not to receive vaccinations. Vaccinations are known triggers for the onset and exacerbation of psoriasis. The effects of vaccinations on us is a great example of how genetic predisposition influences our health. Testing for the presence of the MTHFR gene mutation is now readily available, often with a simple cheek swab. If you seek clarification, ask your health-care provider to order the necessary laboratory test.

We all need methylation pathways to help us detoxify on a cellular level. Individuals with the C677T MTHFR gene mutation have a more difficulty time with detoxification overall, but also particularly with detoxification of metals and metalloids that are often used as adjuvant ingredients in vaccines such as aluminum, arsenic, barium, cadmium, chromium, lead, mercury, selenium, thallium, and zinc.[36]

An *adjuvant ingredient* is one purported to induce the reaction of the immune system to the vaccine.[37]

Being that more than 50 percent of the population have a MTHFR gene mutation that inhibits the body's processing of folic acid and other important B vitamins, if you have psoriasis, I advise you to take a high-quality B complex supplement that includes folate (not folic acid) on a daily basis. In addition, you can request a test for the MTHFR gene.

I grew up taking Tylenol tablets like they were Tic Tacs. The serious risk of acetaminophen-containing drugs for anyone with a MTHFR gene mutation was unknown then, and it is still grossly undiscussed today. Acetaminophen is known to create interference with methylation and detoxification pathways.[38] A person with the MTHFR gene mutation should absolutely stay away from any product containing acetaminophen *especially* in the first three months following a vaccination due to their reduced ability for cellular detoxification through methylation pathways in that timeframe.

Knowing this, it's baffling that pediatricians would routinely recommend to any parents that they give their babies Tylenol to prevent or reduce fevers immediately after vaccination. But for certain, those of us with psoriasis ourselves and those with a family history of psoriasis have to be more careful of toxin exposure in general for themselves and their children. The margin for risking an exposure to all different kinds of substances is simply thinner for us. We must protect our bodies without fail.

Key Cause 4: Emotional Stress

In addition to factors like exposure to toxic chemicals, studies have shown that up to 80 percent of patients experience heightened emotional stress ahead of an autoimmune diagnosis and up to 88 percent of people with psoriasis report emotional stress as a key trigger for their psoriasis. There is also a higher reported incidence of psoriasis in people who experienced a significantly stressful event the previous year, suggesting that stress plays a consequential role in triggering the disease.[39]

Over the years, this has been true for me and for many of the patients I have treated in my practice. During times of high stress, psoriasis does tend to flare up, often significantly. In fact, I can typically intuit the level of emotional stress my patients with psoriasis are feeling simply based on how their skin looks from week to week.

This factor is difficult to weigh in on because . . . let's face it . . . who isn't stressed out these days? Furthermore, when it comes to assessing the stress connection to psoriasis, we all intimately know that coping with psoriasis in and of itself *is* the source of so much of our stress. Stressing about the condition of our skin leads to exacerbation and flareups, which leads to more emotional stress, which of course, results in more outbreaks. Autoimmune conditions follow a vicious cycle.

Although the human body is built to adapt to stress, the extent of chronic stress that we are exposed nowadays can result in the eventuality of maladaptation.

Why Is Our Health Affected So Much by Our Emotions?

We are designed by evolution to have appropriate, healthy responses to high-stress situations. In an emergency, how the nervous system ramps us up works in our favor; in many situations this will be life-saving. When we encounter a stressor, our pupils dilate, our blood pressure goes up, our digestion slows down, and our hormones change. These appropriate, healthy responses to stress enable us to mobilize and flee or fight in order to save our lives or the lives of our loved ones.

Ancestrally, our high-stress situations came in the form of fight, flight, or freeze scenarios like running into a bear in the woods or being chased by a cougar. Although this type of stress could be immense, in the past, danger tended to be short lived. A few hours following the period of high stress, our bodies could return to "normal" and everything returned to being well regulated and relaxed. Back then, a person might have less than five extreme episodes of confronting violent danger in a lifetime.

Nowadays, we sometimes must endure stress for weeks, months, or years. Then, because our bodies aren't meant to withstand chronically stressful conditions, our adaptation mechanisms will become overtaxed. The result is often chronic high blood pressure and chronic digestive problems, like constipation. (Digestion would be placed on hold if we were running from a bear.) As a result of longstanding stress hormone production, cholesterol and blood sugar levels also become chronically elevated. These hormones are intimately connected to cholesterol production and blood sugar pathways. And none of these symptoms occurs by error. Our bodies are responding exactly as they should in the face of stress. The trouble is the duration of the altered biochemistry. Chronic stress might explain why 60 percent of the population (including children) have at least one chronic health condition.[40]

Researchers at Ohio State University School of Medicine investigated how stress affects the speed of healing in the skin (with minor wounds). Skin healing is connected to specific types of hormonal and gene activation. In this study, married couples were given small wounds with suction cups and the level of three proteins involved with skin healing were measured over the course of three weeks.

The couples were asked to have a neutral conversation to establish a baseline. The couples were then instructed to have a conversation that revisited a previous marital argument. When the couples discussed the previous argument, their level of skin healing proteins were suppressed, and in cases where the discussion resulted in significant conflict, the genes responsible for skin and wound healing were downregulated by 40 percent.[41]

Research done with meditation, yoga, mindfulness, and breathing have shown repeatedly that the reverse can also be true. Studies which explore the effects of stress reduction with positive emotions have shown that stress reduction can promote a change in up to 1,561 genes. The change takes place, specifically in genes which up-regulate health and down-regulate stress, as well as with reduced blood pressure and reduced heart and respiration rates. Most of the genetic changes noted were specific to improving the body's response to chronic psychological stresses.

If you spend anytime online, you see all the advice on self-care and the importance of stress management. You might sometimes roll your eyes at the cliché of it all, like I do, thinking, *Tell me something I don't know.*

So, What Are We Supposed to Do about Our Emotional Stress?

Breathwork, yoga, and mindfulness are helpful with stress. I think we all know this. The challenge is that many of us feel like we're spinning our wheels trying to implement another thing and another thing.

When I was in graduate school, a lovely woman named Lynne noticed my psoriasis. She took me aside and suggested that I spend time every day meditating. At this point, I had tried everything, including chemotherapy. But the idea that just sitting still with my legs crossed and my palms up (imagining the lotus position) would help me was confusing—and slightly annoying. Her instruction to "empty your mind and stay in the present" was not workable for me.

In a nutshell, at the time, I simply didn't have the internal bandwidth to make myself available for a commitment to meditation.

That being said, studies suggest there are a number of techniques like meditation that are worth exploring. A systematic review of literature published in 2022 examined nine studies investigating the impact of meditation and mindfulness on psoriasis, quality of life, and symptom severity. All these trials were conducted for eight to twelve weeks. The author of the analysis concluded that in this timeframe mindfulness and meditation definitely can reduce the overall size of the area of psoriasis plaques as well as the severity of the plaquing.[42]

For the purposes of this book, I will focus on a particular few stress-reducing techniques that were life changing for me. Because they feel right and have saved my skin (in every sense), I have permanently welcomed them into my lifestyle. In addition to our discussions of how diet and nutrition, a healthy gut microbiome, and detoxification can improve or even entirely eradicate your psoriasis symptoms, we will explore the power of your mind and of a well-regulated nervous system to help create a healing state.

I plan to take a deep dive into each of the lifestyle techniques I use, during which I will explain why I believe you may find it equally effective for your own situation as I did for mine.

CHAPTER FIVE

Gut Health and the Microbiome

The human microbiome, which is sometimes referred to as our *second genome,* is comprised of diverse, commensal microbes, including bacteria, archaea, fungi, viruses, and parasites that live on our skin, in our lungs and sinuses, in the urogenital tract and vagina (for biological females), and in the GI tract, including both the mouth and the colon. Commensal microbes reside on and in the body and receive nourishment from the foods we eat. In symbiosis with us, they live in harmony with the human body and contribute to the expression of our health in every sense.[1] The entire body is an ecosystem, in fact. It has been estimated that there is one microbiome microbe for every human cell in the body—for a 1:1 ratio.[2]

Within the microbial communities inhabiting different regions of the body, much attention has been drawn to the community residing in the GI tract (gut). The gut, which hosts the densest population of microbes in the body, is colonized by trillions of microorganisms, including bacteria, viruses, eukaryotes (nucleus-containing species), and fungi. The second-most microbially dense area is the skin.[3]

And it just so happens that the gut and the skin are directly connected to each other by the expression of their microbiomes, although the relationship between skin and gut health is a piece of the psoriasis conversation that is often overlooked by health-care providers when they are attempting to cure their patients' psoriasis.

Our personal microbiomes, to a large degree determine how well or poorly we can adapt to our immediate environments, as well as to the entire planet, which has an exceptionally diverse microbiome.

Researchers at the University of California, San Diego, are leading a large-scale, open-source investigation that's being conducted by over 500 collaborators from around the world to create a comprehensive taxonomic map. The Earth Microbiome Project, as it's called, studies the diversity of the soil's microbiome and the planetary microbiome for the benefit of humanity. The underlying value is that we and microbes have a synergistic relationship which bridges our individual health with the health of the planet. Because of the Earth Microbiome Project, our knowledge of our microbial inheritance is rapidly evolving.[4]

What we know already is that an individual's microbiome is an essential component of their immunity and a modifier of the diseases they may experience. It is involved with their personal metabolic, cardiovascular, psychological, and nervous system health. For the purposes of our focus here, we will specifically explore how the human microbiome has been found to be directly correlated to skin diseases, including psoriasis.

Many insults and stresses can damage the composition and function of intestinal microbes. Damage to the life forms living in an individual's gut can come from specific conditions during their birth, the first foods they were given to eat, and their lifelong exposure to stressors including both dietary and environmental toxins.

A baby acquires 100 percent of its primary microbiome from its mother, shortly after conception. This microbiome, which becomes established in utero, can be altered by maternal exposure to drugs and stress and by the quality of the mother's diet and supplementation during the fetus's gestation.[5] It is therefore essential that a prospective mother begins working on balancing her microbiome prior to conception and that she continue to protect and support her microbiome until the birth of her baby. It should be expected that your doctor or midwife be well-versed on the details of how to support and enrich the microbiome throughout pregnancy and immediately prior to giving birth.

Among gut-health experts, a large emphasis is placed on the so-called "first meal," which occurs during birth. As the baby moves through the mother's birth canal (the passageway to the world out of the uterus through the cervix and vagina), it takes in the flora of the mother through its mouth and nasal mucosa. Acquiring maternal flora is so essential to a child's lifelong immunity and adaptation to their environment that, in the event of a C-section delivery, it has become a common practice for obstetric nurses to swab the baby's mouth and nostrils with the mother's birth canal microflora. Ideally, a baby's lifelong microbiome continues to grow and gain internal stability during the first few years of development.

In addition to passing on nutrients, breastfeeding in infancy is also an important way to ensure a diverse and healthy microbiome. Although it is not always possible to breast feed, when it is possible, it is highly preferable. Studies have shown that formula feeding can activate inflammatory pathways that may contribute to autoimmune disease. This theoretically occurs due to early exposure of intact cow's milk protein in formula.[6] Some proteins in human breast milk—oligosaccharides—are prebiotics that nourish healthy gut microbes. Breast milk, in this way, also protects against the development of autoimmunity.[7]

Numerous drugs and toxins can alter our microbiomes during our lifespans. Antibiotics in particular can cause significant and prolonged changes to a microbiome—unintentional harm. Microorganism imbalance (dysbiosis) in the gut occurs despite the best of intentions with antibiotics because, in their targeting, antibiotics cannot differentiate between beneficial and health-threatening bacteria. Although antibiotics can be lifesaving when absolutely necessary, the CDC states that one-third of prescriptions for antibiotics are not needed or are inappropriate. The risk of antibiotic-related damage is heightened for pregnant women as well as babies and children.[8]

Damage to the microbiome and the lining of the gut can result from specific creams, lotions, and topical products coming in contact with the skin. It is important, therefore, for us to ensure that all the topical products we use are protective of the microbiome of the skin. Steroids and other laboratory-made topical products, including creams, makeup, cleansers, and other types of products containing salicylic acid (a significantly damaging ingredient) should be avoided.

Interestingly, biologic therapies used to treat psoriasis appear to have a negative impact on the gut microbiota. Studies have shown that bacterial biodiversity is lower in the guts of participants treated with biologics than in the guts of those who are not.[9]

Furthermore, those who, like me, weren't breastfed as infants, took antibiotics in childhood, have used large amounts of steroids, and have had multiple vaccinations are likely to require deliberate microbiome restoration. The gut microbiomes of healthy subjects differ greatly from the gut microbiomes of people experiencing psoriasis, whose gut health tends to be similar to that of people diagnosed with irritable bowel syndrome.[10]

The good news is that in its natural propensity to heal, the microbiome can recover its balance. It can return to being an enriched environment. Elements in the 90-Day Psoriasis-Healing Program are designed to strengthen the gut microbiome.

Leaky Gut, Autoimmunity, and Psoriasis

The human body evolved to contain highly dynamic and wondrously sophisticated interpretative centers that protect the inside of the body from elements of the outer environment. The skin, the sinuses, and the lining of our intestines can be considered barriers on the "outside" of the body in a sense because they protect the "inside" of us from substances they interpret as foreign or harmful. These membranes separate us from germs, viruses, bacteria, toxic substances, and anything else that lands on us, that we breathe in or which we consume. In real time, these layers of interpretation assimilate information in order to relay proper instructions to our cells, tissues, and organs to help us adapt and ensure our survival.

Any instance in which an interpretive center is bypassed or damaged can result in the body sending up a physiological red flag, in inflammation. If triggering conditions persist, an inflammatory response can go from being acute to becoming chronic in nature. That's the body reporting, "Houston, we've got a problem."

The gut's mucosal lining is semipermeable. This porous quality is necessary to allow water and nutrients to pass through the lining into the bloodstream. Its cells behave like a woven, mesh barrier, perfectly connected by tight junctions. These tight junctions regulate the diffusion of molecules into the bloodstream, by disallowing any molecules larger than a certain size to pass through.[11]

Sometimes, because of inflammatory insults to the gut caused by drugs and toxins, as well as by the kinds of inflammatory foods and nonfoods we previously discussed, the gut lining becomes damaged. The tight junctions then become porous, allowing for larger molecules to pass into the bloodstream, and therefore, into the body. This hyperpermeability is referred to now as *leaky gut syndrome*. Because larger molecules of food particles, like those of wheat and dairy, for example, aren't supposed to enter the bloodstream, the body's immunity and inflammatory pathways are alerted to its undigested presence. Once it's on "high alert," the immune system, recognizing that a foreign material is now interlaced with the bloodstream, can begin to attack the body itself, mistaking it, too, as foreign. This is the phenomenon known as *autoimmunity*.

An ongoing cycle of the body attacking itself is the reason so many people develop autoimmunity, frequently including psoriasis.

Healing the gut is therefore essential for healing psoriasis. In order to heal the gut, we must remove offending foods from our diets, lessen our exposure to toxins, and reduce our stress; and we must also consume whole foods and certain types of food supplements, and establish an optimal, healthy lifestyle.

The Gut–Brain Axis

The gut and the brain are in continuous communication through two long vagus nerves—one on either side of the body—which extend from the brainstem through the neck and into the chest and abdomen. These nerves carry sensory information from the body to the brain, and some of the information they carry comes from the gut. Microbes in the gut help us manufacture chemical transmitters that enable this pathway to function properly. Their quality also contributes to the quality of the messages being exchanged.

The dysbiosis that exists in the guts of people with psoriasis can affect how well the brain functions because it creates an imbalance of the major neurotransmitters and neuromodulators. This can wreak havoc with their moods and their cognition. In part, this explains why people with psoriasis frequently suffer from depression and anxiety.

Although psoriasis itself causes emotional distress—the appearance of plaques that make us self-conscious, the itchiness and burning that interfere with our enjoyment of life—addressing the health of the gut is nonnegotiable because of the evidence showing that the state of the gut is a big factor in our moods. Particularly when we are trying to heal the body, we must acknowledge that the mind and body are directly linked. The brain affects the gut just as much as the gut affects the brain. The gut-brain axis is a two-way street. Knowing of this bidirectional stream of information, we must protect our emotional-attentional space diligently and restore the integrity of the gut.

Both gut healing and emotional healing are necessary elements of my twelve-week-long program.

PART TWO

FOUNDATIONS OF A HEALTHY, WELL-STABILIZED LIFESTYLE

CHAPTER SIX

Inflammatory Foods

"Let food be thy medicine and medicine be thy food."
HIPPOCRATES

We cannot have a conversation about healing psoriasis naturally without a pressing and precise conversation around inflammatory foods and the power of nutrition.

Adopting a lifestyle in which you eat only real, whole fruits, vegetables, and grains, minimally processed and grown as organically and locally as possible, favoring whichever seasonal varieties are available, in a nutshell, is the most healthful way to live. Eating healthy fats, grass-fed meat, and fermented and cultured foods, and eliminating foods that are inflammatory from your diet is easier than it seems, especially when we know *why* to do so.

The 90-Day Psoriasis-Healing Program in this book incorporates the dietary recommendations associated with the well-respected *autoimmune protocol* (AIP).

Although we will be discussing the AIP diet, which I would recommend adhering to strictly for at least twelve weeks, the remainder of the lifestyle I advocate for you and others seeking to heal psoriasis involves reducing your exposure to toxic substances, soothing and regulating your central nervous system, and reprogramming your mind.

This program is not a fad. Not a diet in the sense of attempting to lose weight. I always refer to the guidelines as a *lifestyle* because although there may be a starting line, there will never be a finish line to living as well and naturally as possible. The idea of *dieting* implies impermanence. But ideally, you will embrace these recommendations forever. This lifestyle should be enjoyable and inspiring. As you begin to feel better, you will appreciate the guidelines.

Gone are the days when you and I could eat well for a precise time period only to return to our poor habits once the diet was over. I grew up with a father who routinely told me that he was about to go on another diet and needed to change his habits. He would weave in and out of cabbage soup diets, low-fat diets, low-carb diets, and everything in between. None of them worked for him because they were too restrictive.

Once my father completed a diet, or once he felt burned out on it, he'd simply return to eating his donuts, hot dogs, and store-bought pies. Any weight he took off, he put back on. The seed of truth in his approach was that he knew he needed to change his behavior, he just didn't know how to make healthy nutritional habits sustainable for him.

When I was first looking to make dietary changes to heal my psoriasis symptoms, I remembered my father's behavior and knew I wanted to do something better.

Turning eating well into a sustainable habit requires falling in love with whole foods and food preparation. It also requires us to reorganize our thinking about the values of food beyond physical nourishment, such as how it can bring us together with friends and family. Forming new habits centered on social connection leads to us spending quality time with our loved ones and friends.

When it comes to food preparation: If you are someone who identifies with a "hatred" of the kitchen, I am asking you to allow space in your thinking for curiosity and the possibility of a new beginning. What if you didn't hate cooking? What if cooking could become something you did to relax and calm your mind? What if eating with friends and family became an enjoyable part of your everyday routines?

This is often the juncture in my explanation at which people will say, "I don't even know where to start! Please just give me a list of what to eat and not eat." Rest assured, you will receive instructions. But before we step into the sphere of *"Eat this, not that,"* let's acknowledge that there are many different schools of thought about nutrition, and you may have heard many different opinions in the past. The information in the pages to come is based on my decades of personal experience with psoriasis and with life in general, as well as my professional expertise as a chiropractor.

I identify as a self-proclaimed food and nutrition nerd. Although I was given training on nutrition in graduate school, the way of life I am espousing is founded on thousands of hours of additional review of the scientific research. New information is always coming to light. I hope that my food paradigm and way of life will forever continue to evolve with the best scientific knowledge.

Inflammatory Foods

Psoriasis is associated with chronically elevated blood serum levels of C-reactive protein, interleukins, and cytokines, all of which are markers for inflammation. Inflammation is the root of the problem of autoimmunity; therefore each of us has to ferret out what's causing our own inflammation and make decisions about how best to manage it.

If I was being pressed to name only one culprit in inflammation, I would say *sugar* (tied with seed oils). And if I was also pressed to say one type of food is curative, I'd say *healthy fat*.

We have to be wary of claims made by food companies about the safety of their products and conclusions reached by studies that have been funded by industry—as this is a conflict of interest. On September 12, 2016, the *New York Times* published a brilliant article online entitled "How the Sugar Industry Shifted Blame to Fat."

In it, the writer, Anahad O'Connor divulges that five decades of guidelines (including those which continue to operate today) were founded on the Sugar Association paying off three Harvard scientists back in the 1950s to minimize the link between heart disease (inflammation) and sugar intake and instead to point the finger at fats.[1]

Today, it is understood that fat is an essential nutrient for those of us with psoriasis. We must, however, make sure that we are eating the right kinds of fats and that they are working in our favor as individuals.

I make the following recommendations to my patients experiencing psoriasis.

The Very Rarely or Never Food List

The following foods and ingredients cause inflammation and should be avoided whenever possible.

Processed Grains and Snack Foods

This category includes:

- Packaged baked goods, such as store-bought breads made with enriched flour, oil, and sweeteners

- Breakfast cereal. Most are highly processed and loaded with sugar, and the grains in them are often tainted by pesticides and herbicides.
- Crackers with any kind of hydrogenated oil
- Donuts
- Packaged and boxed muffins, cookies (for example: Twinkies and Oreo cookies)
- Kettle corn, which is most likely GMO, fried, and coated in large amounts of refined sugar.
- Microwaveable popcorn pouches, which are always full of harmful oils and typically use GMO corn.
- Chips
- Processed granola bars: often high in sugars and additives
- String cheese: highly pasteurized and high in sodium
- Puddings and Jell-O: very high in sugar and food coloring

Harmful Oils

This category includes:

- Any product containing hydrogenated or partially-hydrogenated oil. When a hydrogen bond is added to make a liquid oil become a solid at room temperature, the process produces trans fats, which cause intestinal inflammation.

- I Can't Believe It's Not Butter®. This is a blend of vegetables oils disguised as a healthier option to butter. Please note that grass-fed butter is better.
- Nut butters labeled "no stir." In order to prevent the ingredients from separating, harmful emulsifiers and sugars are added to them.
- Fast food. It contains harmful oils and sugars, and is ultraprocessed.
- Deep-fried food. In a restaurant setting, one must assume that the deep fryer oil has been boiling for hours, if not days or weeks. Oils become denatured and inflammatory when heated to such high temperatures, especially for long periods of time.
- Coffee creamers with any flavoring or oils (with the exception of products like Laird Superfood and Four Sigmatic). Creamers are typically artificially flavored and sweetened, and may be high in vegetable oils, like sunflower, soybean, and canola oil, all of which will worsen inflammation.
- Sunflower oil
- Soybean oil
- Peanut oil
- Safflower oil
- Grapeseed oil

Beverages

This category includes:

- Bottled juices, especially those which are pasteurized
- Vitamin waters
- Flavored waters and water-flavoring agents, like packaged lemonade mixes
- Soda. If you like carbonation, stick to seltzer and carbonated waters flavored with organic natural juices.
- Energy drinks of any kind. There are generally proinflammatory due to incorporation of high amounts of added sugar, a dangerously excessive amount of caffeine, and lab-made artificial additives.
- Skim milk or low-fat milk
- Soy beverages. These are highly processed, hormone disruptive, and common triggers for food sensitivity.

See further notes about coffee and wine on page 115.

Dressings, Condiments, and Sauces

This category includes:

- Packaged salad dressing, with the exception of dressing made with olive oil or avocado oil and no artificial ingredients. Store-bought salad dressings typically contain harmful processed oils and large amounts of sugar. Make your own at home instead (*see* recipes on page 195).

- Packaged BBQ sauces, except for paleo, sugar-free, and oil-free sauces, like those sold by companies like Primal Kitchen. Most brands of BBQ sauce are loaded with high-fructose corn syrup or sugar, and food additives like caramel coloring and guar gum (a thickening and stabilizing agent).
- Mayonnaise. Store-bought mayo contains a lot of oil and additives. Instead use mashed avocado, or avocado oil mayonnaise if mayo is absolutely necessary.

Additives and Preservatives

This category includes:

- Aspartame and other artificial sweeteners. Studies show that aspartame causes dysregulation of the gut. It alters our gut's diverse microbial ecology and leads to damage and inflammation.[2]
- Artificial food coloring. Try beet juice, carrot juice, and blueberry juice (or powder) for natural red, orange, and blue food coloring.
- Caramel coloring. This additive is sneaky. It's found in sodas, broths, processed meat, candy, and some vitamins and supplements.

- Carrageenan, a thickener found in alternative milk, heavy cream, ice cream, and yogurt
- Any product labeled "low fat" or "fat free," as these foods are typically high in sugar and harmful thickening agents
- Flavored or sweetened yogurts and kefirs. These products are often high in sugar, food coloring, and thickening agents. These are nothing like true yogurt. For a delicious homemade yogurt recipe, see page 205.
- Products labeled "sugar free" as they are usually artificially sweetened
- Nitrates and nitrites, which are found in cured meats like bacon, ham, hot dogs, cured chorizos, pepperoni, and other sausage, and processed chicken nuggets
- Guar gum, a thickening agent
- Soy sauce, which is high in sodium. Use coconut aminos instead.
- Corn syrup. The corn used is typically genetically modified (GMO) and is highly processed. Corn syrup causes proinflammatory macrophage activation, which dysregulates the gut and perpetuates autoimmunity.[3]
- Frozen meals containing any added harmful oils or sugars
- Farmed fish with food coloring.

Let's take a close look at specific categories of inflammatory foods.

The Nightshades

The nightshade family of plants includes:

- Tomatoes.
- White potatoes.
- Eggplant.
- Okra.
- Peppers.
- Tomatillos.
- Sorrel.
- Gooseberries.
- Ground cherries (with papery husks).
- Pepino melons.
- Paprika.
- Cayenne pepper.
- Capsicum.
- Ashwagandha.

Although all these ingredients are real and can be consumed in an unprocessed form, they do possess certain alkaloids—glycoalkaloids and lectins—that can exacerbate preexisting inflammation and disrupt the mucosal barrier of the gut, making it more permeable. These alkaloids are naturally occurring compounds that may make the food taste bitter or spicy.

During the first six months of your healing journey, I recommend that you consume nightshades only very rarely. This being said, I do not believe that consuming these real and unprocessed foods is the root cause of psoriasis. They are most likely the least of our concerns compared to some of the other "offenders" discussed in this book. In other words, if you have access to a freshly picked, organic tomato, particularly one from your own garden, I suggest that you indulge in every bite of it, but only occasionally. That is, after the first six months of stabilizing your condition.

In a large survey on dietary behavior, with 1,200-people with psoriasis reporting outcomes, 52.1 percent of respondents who eliminated nightshades showed improvements in their symptoms.[4]

Vegetable Oils and Canola Oil

I grew up in a household where canola oil was the exclusive cooking oil in our kitchen. Most of us have a similar history of cooking and baking with canola oil or vegetable oil.

Seed oils, particularly canola oil, are widely used and found in most processed and restaurant-served foods. Canola oil comes from the rapeseed plant, which is in the same family as Brussel sprouts, turnips, and cabbage. Largely produced in Canada, in 1995 the rapeseed plant was genetically modified to withstand the effects of glyphosate in an attempt to aid with large-scale production.

Once again, we are dealing with the gut damage and inflammatory results of eating plants that have been both bioengineered and sprayed with toxic chemicals. It is difficult to locate non-GMO canola oils.[5]

The two main essential fatty acids in our diets are linoleic acid (aka omega 6 fatty acid) and alpha linolenic acid (aka omega 3 fatty acid). These are defined as *essential fatty acids* because our bodies cannot synthesize them; they must be consumed. The reason they are so very important to any conversation about inflammation is that they must be consumed in proper ratios. The current recommend ratio is 4:1. We should consume 1 gram of omega 3s for every four grams of omega 6. If this ratio changes, whether because omega 6 consumption increases or omega 3 consumption decreases, inflammation tends to increase.

According to the U.S. National Institutes of Health, the average American diet presently provides a ratio of 20:1. This is problematic. Where healthy sources of omega 6 come in the form of avocado oil, cashews, peanuts, almonds, and sunflower seeds, the consumption of vegetable oils like soybean oil (ratio of 9:1), corn oil (ratio of 60:1), and safflower oil (ratio of 77:1) can skew the overall ratio in a person's diet. This is why ultraprocessed foods such as chips, packaged baked goods, salad dressings, mayonnaise, fried foods, cereals, and most breads are on the Very Rarely or Never Food List.

Canola oil has a ratio of 2:1 omega-6 to omega-3, which makes it seem as though it would be a good choice. But it most definitely is on the Very Rarely List. The reason? In order to make canola oil, manufacturers use solvents like hexane to extract as much of the oil as possible from the seed. According to the U.S. Environmental Protection Agency (EPA), hexane is a petroleum-based solvent that is a known neurotoxin and proinflammatory agent.

Ninety-five percent of canola oil grown in the United States is genetically modified and also sprayed with herbicides and pesticides. When dealing with an inflammatory condition like psoriasis, it's advisable to do away with it entirely and replace it with coconut oil, extra-virgin olive oil, ghee (clarified butter), and butter. Most brands of canola oil also contain trace amounts of trans fats, which, as mentioned earlier, when we discussed margarine, will trigger inflammation. Studies have shown that vegetable oils like soybean and canola oil will cause inflammation after being consumed for only twenty-eight days.[6]

Because much of the canola oil on the market is found in processed foods and in the kitchen of fast-food restaurants, it's impossible to measure if all of it contains harmful pesticides.

For people experiencing psoriasis, I recommend substituting butter or extra-virgin olive oil for canola oil or vegetable oil in any pie or baked good recipe that calls for one of them. Better safe than sorry.

Furthermore, since canola oil is so commonly used in restaurants, I recommend always asking for your omelet, fried eggs, streaks, meats, and everything in between to be cooked in olive oil or butter. Most restaurants are amenable to this request, particularly if you let them know that you are sensitive to these oils—which is the truth.

The Danger of Glyphosate and Other Herbicides and Pesticides

Glyphosate is a chemical infamously found in the herbicide Roundup, originally manufactured by Monsanto but now made by Bayer after a $66 billion-dollar corporate merger took place in 2018. Roundup has been the subject of thousands of legal actions, and it is still on sale years later despite what science has shown about how deadly it can be. Exposure has been linked to non-Hodgkins lymphoma, for example.[7]

Genetically modified organisms (GMOs) are plants modified in a lab in order to aid in the survival of the seed when exposed to the chemicals contained in pesticides like Roundup. This was developed for the sake of mass agriculture, so farmers could spray an entire field of crops with Roundup, thereby killing all the weeds without killing the plant being grown for consumption.

Through this process, glyphosate, the active pesticide in Roundup, makes its way into the plant and eventually onto our plates. Glyphosate is the world's most extensively used agrochemical. It is now estimated that we spray more than 4.5 billion pounds of glyphosate on crops, which leeches into the soils, plants, and water systems of our planet. And there are now dozens of genetically modified plant species around the world that have allowed chemical companies to develop a seemingly infinite market for their weedkillers.

Foods labeled "non-GMO" sound like a healthy, safe alternative, but unfortunately this is smoke in mirrors. The "non-GMO" label seems to imply that these foods are free from glyphosates, but although the seeds are free of genetic modification, the crops may still be vastly exposed to products like Roundup before it is time for harvest. In other words, the non-GMO designation is not synonymous with "chemical free."

Non-GMO foods, particularly grains, tend to be sprayed with Roundup to accelerate crop cultivation. Farmers have often had difficulty getting wheat and barley to dry evenly in order to start harvesting them efficiently. To expedite the preharvest timeline, Roundup is sprayed to kill the crop, thereby accelerating the drying of the grain. This method is either called *late harvest spraying* or *crop desiccation.*

It is well documented that glyphosates alter the microbes in our gastrointestinal tracts, and as we will discuss in the next chapter, if we degrade our microbiomes, we lose healthy and necessary communication at the skin level, which reduces the regenerative potential of our skin.

Studies indicate that exposure to glyphosates, through microbiome alteration, creates proinflammatory cytokines—small, protein-based signaling molecules in the immune system—which is the opposite effect than that which we require when we're trying to heal from psoriasis. The literature references a link between glyphosate exposure and the actual triggering of psoriasis, not to mention neurodegenerative disorders like Alzheimer's disease.[8]

The foods we eat, as much as possible should be organic (chemical-free), and ideally regeneratively farmed. By law, organic foods cannot be sprayed with glyphosate or any other insecticide or herbicide.

It appears that we share a microbiome with the planet. All organisms contribute to the richness and balance of this microbiome. The health of our personal microbiomes is reflected in the health of the microbiome of the soil. The health of our microbiomes is also intricately connected to the health of livestock and wild animals, plants, fungi, pollinators, and the rest of the planetary biosphere.[9]

Regenerative farming practices have been shown to be an answer to soil desiccation and other types of damage caused by mass agriculture, and doing our part by choosing to lead a glyphosate-free lifestyle not only can help us heal as individuals but it will also promote the regeneration of our soil, waterways, and air.

Particularly, watch out for the following foods, which are red flagged for glyphosate contamination.

Please note that the foods listed in the box on the next page are generally thought of as healthy choices, but when tainted by glyphosates, they become more reactive and inflammatory.

Watch Out for the Following Glyphosate-Laden Foods

Granolas made by Quaker, KIND, Back to Nature, and Nature Valley
Instant oats made by Giant, Quaker, Umpqua, and Market Pantry
Whole oats made by Quaker, Bob's Red Mill, Nature's Path, and 365 Whole Foods Markets
Cereal by Kashi and Kellogg's (Lucky Charms, Cheerios, and Honey Nut Cheerios)
Snack bars made by Quaker, KIND, Nature Valley, and Kellogg's
Orange juice by Tropicana, Minute Maid, Signature Farms, and Kirkland
Crackers, including Cheez-Its, Ritz, Triscuits, Goldfish
Cookies made by Annie's, Kashi, and Nabisco (Oreo cookies)
Chips made by Stacy's, Frito-Lay (Lay's, Doritos, Fritos)
Almonds (unless organic)
Beets (unless organic)
Beet sugar (unless organic)
Carrots (unless organic)
Quinoa (unless organic)
Vegetable oil (unless organic)

CHAPTER SEVEN

Psoriasis-Healing Foods

The following foods are encouraged; please eat them in as much varietal combination as possible. Eating foods that are in season and grown close to your home is a best practice because freshness matters. Becoming acquainted with local farmers and shopping at farmers markets in your town will help you to develop a relationship with the produce you eat and to become connected to the quality of the soil it has grown in. Expecting to have access to information on pesticides and handling of plant foods isn't realistic in a typical grocery store setting, whereas small farmers tend to have a strong appreciation for healthy soil and an intimate connection with their crops.

Outside of big cities, most communities now have ready access to organic produce grown on small, local farms that participate in seasonal community supported agriculture (CSA) programs where consumers can sign up for a seasonal fresh-food subscription. The enrollment fee is paid in advance to help the farm cover seed costs and labor to get planting underway. If you participate, then once a week you can pick up a box containing vegetables and fruits—and some CSA farms offer eggs, dairy, fish, and meat, too. This is a great way to eat produce from local soil and to form a trusting relationship with organic farmers.

See the Resources at the back of the book for information on how to find a CSA program near you.

I love challenging myself to eat forty different plant foods per week during growing season, including fruits, vegetables, legumes, herbs, sprouts, nuts, and seeds. This wonderful way to boost creativity around meals has profound health benefits.

The Eat This Food List below is a very specific guide to foods that will inflammation in check and nourish the gut and bodily tissues. I encourage you to try all of the foods on this list. These foods, barring any to which you have sensitivities or allergies, are meant to be eaten as a way of life for the rest of your life once you have completed the 90-Day Psoriasis-Healing Program. They will help you to stabilize your condition and maintain good health going forward.

The Eat This Food List

The following categories and lists of foods should be implemented at will, providing that you focus both on variety itself, and on trying a variety of foods that you may not have previously considered. Being creative with cooking styles and different combinations of ingredients will offer you endless possibilities.

Healthy Fats

Most of us were sold the lie that oils should be avoided because all fat was hazardous to heart health and would cause inflammation. Although this is true of some oils, like canola (rapeseed) oil, which we covered in Chapter 6, those who follow the Mediterranean diet and most of the centenarians living in the so-called Blue Zones—places where folks have extraordinary longevity—make use of generous amounts of fresh olive oil.

A properly chosen olive oil is a superfood that has been shown to decrease inflammation, stabilize blood glucose, promote heart health, aid in the betterment of mental health, and lower cancer rates, as well as all-cause mortality. The polyphenols found in abundance in olive oil, avocado oil, and walnut oil are powerful antioxidants which specialize in repairing cellular damage. They inhibit inflammatory enzymes and reduce the production of inflammatory cytokines.[1]

Oxidation—the forming of free radical molecules—can occur when we heat oils to high temperatures; but because the fat molecules in olive oil are double bonded, it is subject to less oxidation than other oils. While olive oil is great to cook with, it's also delicious eaten raw over a salad or drizzled on top of food. For these reasons, it is the first of our sources of healthy fats.

- Olive oil. The best olives oils to buy are younger, first cold-pressed, extra-virgin olive oils. These oils have not undergone rigorous processing other than being spun in a centrifuge to separate them from the solid residues and water in olives and simply being pressed. (*See* Resources for the name of my favorite olive oil club.)
- Coconut oil. It has a higher smoke point than olive oil and is a good choice for cooking.
- Butter made from the milk of grass-fed cows and goats
- Ghee, a style of clarified butter that's great for those with dairy sensitivities
- Coconut oil
- Duck fat
- Beef tallow
- Fish, especially salmon
- Beef from grass-fed cows
- Eggs from pasture-raised chickens
- Pastured chicken
- Sardines (canned in water or extra-virgin olive oil)
- Organ meat
- Bone broth from mammals and poultry
- Plain yogurt made from whole milk (not low fat) that comes from grass-fed cows
- Cultured dairy products like sour cream, crème fraîche, and kefir

- Hard, white, aged cheeses like parmesan and Manchego
- Raw nuts, especially macadamias
- Hemp seeds
- Flax seeds
- Chia seeds

Healthy Grains and Breads

Grains and breads have a bad reputation for causing inflammation and with good reason. Throughout the twelve weeks of my program, it will be beneficial to eliminate grain from your diet. However, once your health condition has been stabilized, you can reintroduce grain. From then on, don't let it scare you, as it can be cooked nourishingly and deliciously. You just have to be clever about it.

In order to ensure the nourishing integrity of the grain you consume, you may have to get a bit "nerdy" about it. Starting with grain in its whole form (as opposed to its processed form, or as flour) is advisable. Try cooking grains like einkorn, emmer, barley, and farro the same way as you would prepare rice—by soaking it first, before heating it. You'll find "Instructions for Soaking and Sprouting Dry Grains, Beans, and Legumes Before Cooking" on page 110. These grains taste a bit nutty and have a wonderful texture. Sourcing your organic, whole grains that are grown on smaller farms is ideal. (*See*

Resources for ideas about finding organic grain farms to order from.)

I wholeheartedly believe that bread can and should be an essential part of sharing food as a family because "breaking bread" together can bring us together emotionally. Bread was one of the staples of our early ancestors, and I believe that with the right grain and right conditions and preparation, bread can become a superfood which nourishes us and deepens our connection to others.

The bread sold in most grocery stores today is bastardized from its origins—so much so, in my opinion, that it really shouldn't be called *bread.* A general rule of thumb should be not to eat store-bought bread or packaged bread of any kind.

But we're here now to talk about the delicious foods that you *can* eat! A sourdough loaf made with a fresh flour made from heirloom grains, such as spelt, emmer, einkorn, or red winter wheat, and which has been fermented for twelve to sixteen hours, or even longer, is a completely different matter.

The fermentation in sourdough is said to contribute immensely to the health of our gut microbiomes by introducing enzymes and beneficial organisms. The fermentation process also changes the structure of the grain by predigesting it, thereby greatly reducing its gluten content, which makes the bread more nutrient dense and less likely to be reactive. (*See* my favorite long-ferment, whole-grain sourdough bread recipe, on page 202.)

If you're someone who loves bread and could really get into this, I recommend milling grain yourself on the days you'll be making bread. (At home, I use a wooden KoMo hand-cranked grain mill.) Search online for places where you can buy whole grain either in sacks or from a store near you. Some people love the idea of milling grain at home, and others think the suggestion is very much "over the top." I understand both perspectives.

If baking bread at home is not an option for you—or you would prefer never to have it become an option—try to find a nearby bakery that makes an organic whole-grain, long-fermented sourdough (often called *levain)* bread. After eating a loaf or two, see how it makes you feel and assess how well you tolerate it.

Occasionally, instead of doing my own baking, I buy Ezekiel bread, which contains sprouted grains. (This is found in the freezer section of health-food stores or in the health-food aisles of regular supermarkets.) Everything about it is wonderful, with the exception that the bread makers add gluten to the final product (most unfortunate).

Our list of healthy grains and breads includes:

- Brown rice.
- Sprouted grain breads (only from the freezer section, and only if there are no added sugars or oils).
- True sourdough breads (long ferments).
- Spelt.
- Quinoa. Should be soaked and rinsed to remove *saponins,* antinutrients that protect the plant from

being digested by other organisms. Saponins are soapy tasting and also can be used as a soap. For this reason, some people recommend reserving the quinoa soaking water for use as a hair rinse. (*See* "Instructions for Soaking and Sprouting Dry Grains, Beans, and Legumes" on page 110.)

- Barley.
- Emmer.
- Einkorn.
- Rye.

Healthy Sources of Fiber

Short-chain fatty acids, namely butyrate, propionate, and acetate, are beneficial metabolites produced in the gut when we consume fiber from various sources, including:

- Whole grains (left intact and not ground into flour).
- Nuts.
- Avocados.
- Berries.
- Beans and other legumes, such as pulses (lentils and chickpeas), peas, and peanuts. Legumes are plants whose fruits are pods that contain seeds. They're incredibly healthy because they are low in cholesterol and high in fiber and protein.

The presence of these short-chain fatty acids is directly related to the health and diversity of microbes in the gut microbiome. Research shows that they are both anti-inflammatory for the gut and also for the skin because of improving the functioning of the epithelial (skin cell) barrier.[2]

Being that many of us were taught that grains and legumes can lead to inflammation in the gut, I can see how this conflicting information may require a change of thinking on our parts. It's also confusing because, during the cleansing phase of the AIP diet, we're told to eliminate grains and legumes from our meals entirely.

I do believe that the AIP diet is effective in healing psoriasis, and sometimes very necessary, *but I don't* believe that restrictions on grains and legumes should be needed in the long term. Eliminating grains and legumes makes sense for the duration of my ninety-day program, but once you transition back to a more diverse diet, implementing whole grains and legumes should be beneficial to your microbiome.

We also get healthy fiber from:

- All vegetables.
- All fruits.
- All fresh herbs like parsley, cilantro, oregano, basil, dill, and tarragon.
- All squashes.

INSTRUCTIONS FOR SOAKING AND SPROUTING DRY GRAINS, BEANS, AND LEGUMES

Soaking dry grains, beans, and legumes in water mixed with two to three tablespoons of whey or plain yogurt is a simple and effective lacto-fermentation technique that helps make these fibrous foods more easily digestible. When grains and beans and other legumes are dried, they form protective barriers around them referred to as *antinutrients,* which in essence render them undigestible to any bird or animal that might consume them. The antinutrient properties of the dried grain or legume increase its chance of passing through the creature's digestive system, in whole form, hence giving it a chance to sprout once it lands on soil again. It is a self-preservation method.

Soaking dry grains, beans, and legumes renders them more easily digestible, and provides for a better absorption and utilization of nutrients. This decreases inflammation and irritation to the gut.

SOAKING. To soak, simply place the amount of dry grain, beans, or legumes to be used in a large mason jar, and fill it with water and a tablespoon or two of whey or yogurt. Allow it to sit for six to ten hours, or overnight. Rinse well and cook as you normally would.

If you wish, at this point you can also sprout the plant. This conveniently transforms the dried grain or legume into a much

more bioavailable plant with higher levels of vitamin C and more enriched and complete B vitamin ratios.

SPROUTING. If you wish to go further and sprout the grain, beans, or legumes, rinse them thoroughly and simply place the previously soaked grain, bean, or legume in a jar with a screen lid or a layer of cheese cloth across the mouth. Rinse the contents thoroughly three times per day and afterward place the jar upside down in a bowl or tray for proper drainage. If the jar doesn't have good drainage, the contents will become sludgy and they will not sprout properly.

Once you see small sprouts, cook the grain, bean, or legume as you would in its dried form, but please note that the cooking time will be reduced because the grain, bean, or legume is now softer, being that it has become a living plant again.

I have found that sprouted grains and legumes taste fresher and somehow more complex and delicious.

The Weston Price Foundation discusses soaking, fermenting, and sprouting in detail in Sally Fallon's brilliant book *Nourishing Traditions.*

Other Nutrient-Rich Foods That Are Healing

The following foods, which are considered superfoods, can be added to other foods and recipes to enhance their nutrient density and healing factors.

Seaweed

Making regular use of dried seaweeds, which are naturally high in iodine and rich in minerals, can easily become a super healthy kitchen habit. Dried and powdered seaweed can be added to soups, stews, and sauces, lending itself as an effortless and nutritious way to implement the superfood into weekly cooking.

Mushrooms

Mushrooms are particularly high in vitamin D and offer excellent immune system support. You can eat them in salads, soups, rice dishes, and stews. Another seamless way to consume some mushrooms daily is to procure a powdered blend that can be mixed into your morning coffee. If you don't love whole mushrooms, this way is good camouflage. (*See* Resources for brand recommendations.)

Fruit Smoothies and Juices

A packaged smoothie can have as much sugar as a can of soda. For example, an Odwalla Strawberry Banana juice has 41 grams of sugar vs. 39 grams of sugar in a standard can of Coca-Cola. Also, beware of any smoothie made from any type of concentrate. Many strip mall and airport smoothie establishments will use orange juice made from concentrate as the base for their smoothies, but concentrate tends to be very high in sugar, and therefore, it is proinflammatory.

By contrast, you can enjoy fresh, homemade smoothies and freshly pressed juices (*see* Chapter 12 for recipes). I personally love a good, fresh-pressed juice. My favorite is the Turmeric Lemon Ginger Shots on page 209. If you're going to invest in a juicer for home use, look for a slow-masticating juicer like the GreenStar.

Making your own smoothies at home is a good way to boost your intake of fiber from fruits and vegetables; as well as protein, by adding nut butters or grass-fed whey; and healthy fat by incorporating a tablespoonful of extra-virgin olive oil or coconut oil.

Supergreen Powders

Supergreen powders come in many varieties and brands. I prefer those that are organic and freeze-dried, like Green Vibrance® or AG1®. Ideally, yours will offer the nutrients of numerous, diverse plants, including greens, yellows, and purples from sources that include sea vegetables (kelp) and grasses.

My advice is to find one whose flavor you like (or can tolerate). AG1 has a slight taste of pineapple and vanilla. This is not my "cup of tea," but it may be yours.

The best supergreen powders also contain digestive enzymes and diverse probiotics, including strains of Lactobacillus, Bifidobacterium, and Streptococcus, which can help restore the health of a compromised gut microbiome.

Supergreen powders can be added to a smoothie or juice, or just to a glass of water. When I make mine, I juice a half grapefruit or orange with a citrus hand juicer, then mix in my supergreen powder, and I drink them right out of the juice-capturing cup. This simplifies the whole process by eliminating an extra dish.

Anyone with digestive troubles, including constipation and/or acid reflux and heartburn, should definitely consider supplementing their diet with supergreen powder. Being that gut repair is at the forefront of our psoriasis-healing journey, these greens are an easy place to start. They can be a great help with regularity and digestion. (*See* Resources section.)

Fermented Foods

Fermented foods like sauerkraut and kimchi can be worked into your weekly diet by eating a dollop here and there along with your meals. Fermentation occurs thanks to the presence of beneficial bacteria (probiotics) that aid with digestion and building balance in the gut microbiome. I like to use them as a sort of condiment or small side dish.

Particularly when fermented in your own space—because your home has a unique microbiome—sauerkraut and kimchi can help restore the health of your gut, thereby reducing inflammation. (*See* the recipe for sauerkraut on page 197.)

Red Wine (But Only One to Two Glasses at a Sitting)

If like me, you're a fan of wine, seek out a wine that is sugar-free and farmed organically. Look for wines that have a lower-than-average alcohol content, lower sulfites, are produced on small family farms, and are dry farmed (meaning, grown without irrigation).

How can a wine be sugar free if it is made from fruit? Because if you do not disrupt its natural processes, the yeast involved with wine fermentation consumes all the sugar from the grapes once the wine is in the bottle aging. Sugar-free wines are robust and delicious, just not as sweet as some mass-produced vintages you may be accustomed to drinking.

It is estimated that only 5 percent of wines are truly organic. Unfortunately, as of 2016, glyphosate was found in 100 percent of the California wines samples tested, including some wines that were labeled organic.

Things are not better in France. In 2017, Emmanuel Macron, then the president of France, began the process of eliminating glyphosate from French agricultural practices. This caused an uproar and the powers that be then extended the allowable use of glyphosate on crops until 2033. One can assume that French wines are likely to be glyphosate-contaminated.[3]

As of May 2023, the following wine-producing countries instituted restrictions on glyphosate. I like to seek out small-batch wineries from these countries.

- Argentina (partial ban)
- Austria (partial ban)
- Italy (complete ban)
- Spain (complete ban)

Finding clean, unaltered wine is difficult. For this reason, I am a big advocate and subscribing member of Dry Farm Wines, a company that does the research for its customers and hand-selects wines from vineyards and wineries committed to small batches of organic, irrigation-free, sugar-free, and low-sulfite wines. (*See* Resources for details on contacting them.)

Coffee, Tea, and Kombucha

Anyone who reads the research on coffee will have their mental marbles rolling with confusion. Or maybe it's just me. I have spent years deeply investigating coffee because *I love coffee*. From what I've deciphered personally, by reading the research and keeping an open mind while considering the remarks of pro-coffee and anti-coffee pundits, is the following: Like almost anything else, coffee can be toxic or it can be a superfood. It's just that, with coffee, because most of us drink it daily, it can lead to the accumulation of toxicity in our bodies very quickly.

Conventional brands of coffee (think Folgers and Starbucks) are among the most heavily chemically treated food products in the world. Some of the chemicals used are unstable in heat and thus disappear after roasting, but others, like glyphosate, linger.

The coffee pods used in machines like Keurig are typically plastic, and it is well known that microplastics are disruptive to the gut microbiome. There are also studies suggesting that microplastics can disrupt the normal function of immune cells, leading to an immune response characteristic of autoimmunity.[4] So, you want to avoid brewing coffee in pods, too. Bad coffee made in a bad way is a double whammy of gut disruption.

When looking for coffee, look for certified organic brands that are tested to ensure they are free of pesticides, molds, mycotoxins, and other contaminants. Some coffees are formulated to offer rich antioxidant properties, and some are specifically formulated for digestive health. (*See* Resources for a list of my favorite coffees.)

Herbal teas like chamomile, peppermint, dandelion root, turmeric, and ginger are acceptable. Please note that the standards on teas and their toxicity levels are very poor, so you should go out of your way to find the highest quality organic herbal teas possible.

When it comes to tea, also do your best to avoid the microplastics in synthetic teabags. Either brew loose-leaf tea or brew tea presented in an unbleached, paper tea bag.

Kombucha is a fermented tea filled with probiotics and antioxidants that has a pleasing zing to it. Drunk cold, that slight fizziness makes it a heathier alternative than drinking soda. Just be cautious about the amount of sugar in the bottle. Some brands are loaded with sugar, which, as you know, is proinflammatory.

Healing Superfoods to Integrate with Your Regular Nutrition Habits

- Pickles
- Garlic
- Bee pollen
- Honey
- Cacao
- Dark chocolate (70 percent or higher)
- Dried fruit (without added sugar or oils)
- Ginger
- Fresh herbs (lots)
- Spices (lots, including turmeric)
- Raw apple cider vinegar (*see* recipe on page 200)
- Marine collagen (types 1 and 3)—add to soups
  - Sea salt or Real® salt

CHAPTER EIGHT

The Healing Power of Your Mind

The human body will always have a propensity for healing. If we create optimal conditions for healing and remove obstacles, healing becomes the natural default system. Our body's innate intelligence, however, relies as much on the way we think as it does every other aspects of our lifestyles. And for many of us, the way we think is often the overlooked elephant in the room.

As I slowly educated myself on the various causes of psoriasis and what worked and didn't work for me, on autoimmune health, gut health, nutrition, supplementation, inflammation, and all the *dos* and *don'ts* of an optimally healthy lifestyle, I became hyperfocused (to put it lightly) on my healing project.

Focus can be a wonderful thing. It is the mental equivalent of a platform for diving into a swimming pool-sized quantity of research and experimentation head first.

Focusing intently enables us to put our blinders on and to direct all of our attention on the task in front of us. For me, however, it became excessive; and looking back on it now, I can see that my behavior became obsessive.

During the time of my life when I was learning how to heal my psoriasis, bit by bit, the healing project began to dictate everything I did, and even more dramatically, everything I didn't do. The self-imposed restrictions were severe. I became vegetarian, then a raw vegan. I eliminated dairy, then sugar. I stopped chewing gum. I stopped eating bread and wheat products. I stopped drinking coffee and eliminated alcohol from my diet with the exception of an occasional glass of red wine.

For some people, making such lifestyle changes would be a no-brainer. Your own internal response to my admission, in fact, may be, *Well, yes, of course it's what you should do. What's the problem?* But for me, the inflexible way of being I was adopting felt like a box I had squeezed myself into. The box gradually shrank until it was so small that I couldn't move and could barely breathe without fear of what would happen if I didn't find a way to make the box even smaller. I was that scared of what my skin would do on a minute-to-minute basis.

If I was invited somewhere for dinner or to a pool party in the afternoon and the hosts were serving something like pizza, I believed that I would have to choose between "being rude" and not eating ("starving" myself) or accepting the gracious offering along with the expectation, the knowing, that I would wake up the next morning with worse skin than the day before. I would stress about every morsel that went into my mouth, convinced that if the "wrong" choice was made I would pay for it and suffer the punishment of skin on fire the next day. I believed it would all happen because I had dared to leave the box.

I would wake up in the morning and take a reluctant look at myself, hoping for a miracle. Every morning, facing the absence of an apparently impossible miracle, I would beat myself up for not doing enough and not "following through" enough on my self-imposed rules.

Where my husband, children, and I ate, what we ate, how we went out, and everything in between was dictated by my fear and obsessive commitment to avoidance. When people around me expressed concern for my behavior and lack of patience, it created tension and I became frustrated. I felt that nobody understood my situation, and it was true. Nobody understood.

In other words, I was a lot of fun to be with.

I have since come to learn that the health paradigm in which I was raised views the human body as a compartmentalized system. The stomach is seen as separate from the liver, which is separate from the heart, which is separate from the pancreas, which is separate from the skin, which is separate from the gums, which is separate from the thyroid, and so on. This paradigm expects our body parts to be treated individually and separately.

Today, I am aware that everything in the body is connected and intertwined, and that the mind and body are not only entirely connected but are influencing one another in real time without pause. But back then, I was just learning that the gut and skin have a direct relationship. The idea that my thoughts are directly related was something I didn't yet comprehend.

Over the years, I had heard philosophical adages like "Form follows energy," "You are what you think you are," and "I think, therefore I am." Coming from a culture of embodied separation, wherein all physical parts are considered independent, to me, the mind–body connection was something that only members of the yoga community and Buddhists talked about. Healing my body by changing my thinking felt too farfetched and "woo-woo" for someone like me who believes in science. And *I literally had already tried everything else and failed.*

I had been studious and scientific about my health condition and sought out the experts, the ones with impressive credentials working in posh offices with frosted glass doors and marble countertops. It certainly wasn't going to be my mind that was the missing link—no way.

I can't recall how I came upon the book *The Secret* by Rhonda Byrne, just that I read it in a single afternoon, like I was inhaling my first breath of fresh air after being imprisoned in a stagnant, windowless room. The book made me look up from my hyperfocus. It was a pattern disruptor for my intelligent, educated mind.

Although the book itself isn't spectacularly written, the content isn't referenced, and it is a bit fluffy and ethereal, reading it shone a light for me on the quality of my thinking. In so doing, it served as a catalyst to change my approach. But first I had to get past the unpleasantness of discovering what I found when I started paying attention to what my mind had been telling my body for years.

Nothing to Lose

It was in the summer of 2008, at the age of thirty-three, when, for the first time in my life, I slowed down and looked, listened, focused, and paid attention to my thoughts—to what I was telling myself about myself. Nobody had ever taught me that my thoughts were connected to anything in particular, let alone my health or my entire life for that matter before.

My boys were three and five year old then, meaning I had been tirelessly working toward healing for over ten years and been a psoriasis sufferer for twenty-one years. The box I lived in was nailed shut by the thousands of restrictive rules I'd imposed on myself out of fear that things would get worse.

I had flown back east with my two boys, to Ontario, Canada, for the wedding of a cousin. The ceremony was to take place on my parents beautiful one-hundred-acre property on the Ottawa River, in farm country. The three of us had flown in six days early and my husband, Darin, would be arriving later. I had just read *The Secret* prior to arriving and was intrigued by the prospect of taking a look at my thoughts. I was curious. I could hear an intuitive whisper telling me that I needed to look inside—and I mean *deeply look*, unabashedly and unafraid.

The return to my busy life as a business owner, chiropractor, wife, mother, community member, and everything else was to occur in eight days. My parents were with me and in love with my boys, so I saw the week before the wedding as a valuable opportunity to explore my inner world. Other than Darin, only my parents intimately knew my suffering in regard to my psoriasis, and as any parent would, they suffered with it also. When I shared my curious notion and desire to "take a look" with them, they gave me emotional support for me and agreed to provide attentive care to my kids, for five days in a row.

For each of those five summer days, I took a walk down a beautiful country road alongside the river, trekking about fifteen to twenty kilometers there and back without a phone or any other potential distraction. For the hours that the walk took, I focused on simply observing my thoughts. *What am I telling myself,* I wondered?

Over the first and second day, I noticed that every few minutes, if not every few seconds, but certainly not less than every two to three minutes, I was unrelentingly thinking about my skin. Furthermore, the subconscious, barely noticeable disparaging language I was using to speak with myself was shocking and heartbreaking. I could feel, in my gut and in my heart, that this constant self-berating stream of thought was connected to why I was so "stuck" with my healing. I had an intuitive sense that this was why, despite doing all the right things with my physical health, there was no change. The physical had been more than handled.

Looking back at it, I now believe that the extensive physical work I was doing to support my body stood no chance against the thousands of self-criticizing thoughts I was replaying in my mind minute by minute and day after day. Thoughts like: *I'm ugly, I'm disgusting, I look like a lizard, I should hide, I'm gross, I bet it's worse now, now—is it worse?* and on and on, were sabotaging any hope for my healing.

I couldn't believe it. How had I not been aware that I was doing this? I knew that I was stressed, that my self-esteem was poor, and that I wanted a new birthday suit, *but how could I be using such derogatory language to speak to myself?*

It's amazing how the tapes that are stuck on repeat in our minds can turn into background noise and be tuned out while we're frantically looking everywhere else for the answer to the question of what ails us. But whether or not we know it our hearts—and guts—are undistractedly plugged into the inner monologue.

Here is how my week progressed.

I spent the first day just observing, trying not to judge the noise in my head or myself. I was just noticing the thoughts that came up.

The second day, I began working on catching every self-deprecating thought and flipping it on the spot to an opposite thought, like: *I'm beautiful; My skin is smooth, pearly, and silky; I'm so grateful for this beautiful life and this beautiful skin;* or *My skin is so soft and healthy, it looks flawless.* I would try to elicit a feeling of gratitude in my heart and from my heart along with my new thoughts.

Also, I visualized myself naked, standing in front of a full-body mirror looking clear-skinned and in love with how beautiful I was and how much I loved myself. I pretended that I had never had a skin issue at all, not for a moment. That none of my symptoms or upset had ever existed and that a heart-driven love for myself was all I had needed. I reinvented myself, right there on that beautifully winding road, which smelled like hay, wildflowers, and manure.

On the third day, shifting my thinking became exhausting because I felt as if I was having to lie to myself over and over, and I had to believe the lies. Then it occurred to me that maybe I'd been lying to myself for years and my new thought pattern was actually the truth.

I was still thinking several negative thoughts per minute at points that day, so I had the opportunity to diligently rehearse the new, better thoughts over and over and over for hours while I walked.

On day four, I began experiencing a new sense of certainty about the importance of reinventing my story. I had the unexplainable feeling that this was the most powerful thing I had ever done. I was energized and felt hopeful. I was working on my mind every second I could get.

My parents continued to be supportive of my solo activity, and if they had any skepticism or concern that their daughter was off her rocker, they (thankfully) hid it well. By the end of that day, my skin began to clear; it was happening in front of my eyes, in real time, hour by hour—just like that.

By the fifth day, I had reinvented how I saw myself. I was overcome with gratitude for the beautiful skin I live in. The painful past no longer existed. I felt recharged and open instead of contracted and consumed. I had mended whatever was broken in me. The healing was complete.

When my husband arrived, his amazement and disbelief over the physical, emotional, and spiritual transformation that I'd undergone in less than a week can only be explained by saying that he was witnessing a miracle. That day, my skin was completely clear and having been through the entire journey together, the only thing left was gratitude.

Eighteen years later, I have never—not even for a moment—had another struggle with psoriasis, and I have faith that I never will. The problem has been transcended. For the first ten years after my skin healed, I didn't talk about psoriasis at all because I couldn't allow it to be part of my ongoing reality—not even as part of my past. Once I felt safe talking about healing my thinking, however, I realized that my story could be helpful to others. Now I believe that it is part of my purpose to share the story.

I continue to practice daily affirmations expressing gratitude for my health and well-being, and for my healing. These sound something like: "Thank you for my beautiful skin. Thank you for my health. Every day, in every way, I am getting better and better. I open my heart to abundant health, inspiration, beauty, and creativity, and these come to me easily and naturally like water flowing down a hillside. With faith and belief in a splendid life, I know that I am a miracle."

I can imagine how fantastical this anecdote might sound. I understand why the internal component of healing psoriasis that I espouse could seem impossible or unrealistic, particularly to those who have taken every prescription medication, applied every topical cream and steroid, and also unbelievably simplistic to those who have spent thousands on supplements, enemas, tanning beds, and everything in between without getting the results they sought.

I've had numerous conversations with people who cannot bring themselves even to entertain the possibility that the power of their thoughts in combination with the power of their hearts may in the end be the most important pieces in their healing puzzle. My response is always the same: "What if what I'm sharing with you is your missing link?"

The Placebo Effect

Harvard-educated surgeon and anesthesiologist Henry Beecher, M.D., worked in field hospitals during World War II. At the time, there were so many patients in crisis from needing amputations and other unimaginably painful, invasive procedures that it was common to run out of morphine. Beecher reported that he'd witnessed a nurse, out of desperation, tell a patient that she was injecting him with morphine, though it was saline, and in a matter of minutes, he wasn't feeling any pain. This enabled the patient to have a pain-free amputation.

Impressed by what he'd seen time and time again, Beecher began giving saline injections to soldiers who believed they were receiving morphine, and then would perform extensive surgeries without any reports of pain. His successful experiences with this technique drove him to study the phenomenon now known as the *placebo effect* extensively once he returned home to the United States. He published a clinical review of fifteen studies in *The Journal of the American Association* that prompted the scientific model for medical research resulting in what we now refer to as randomized, controlled trials. In such trials, placebos are used randomly so that they do not interfere with test results.[1]

Historical documentation of the alteration of physical reality through the use of thoughts dates all the way back to the Bible with its many stories of miraculous healing.

In 2010, Ted Kaptchuk, O.M.D., professor of global health and social medicine at Harvard University and the director of the Harvard-wide Program in Placebo Studies and the Therapeutic Encounter at Beth Israel Deaconess Medical Center in Boston, Massachusetts, astonishingly showed that placebos work, even when people know that they are taking a placebo. This outcome was specifically tested on participants with IBS who received a bottle labeled "placebo pills." The participants transparently understood that they were taking a "sham treatment" so they weren't being tricked into anything, yet only three weeks into the study, participants who received the placebo reported twice as much relief as participants receiving no treatment.[2]

Over the years, I have observed that during times of high stress for me and countless patients of mine, psoriasis tends to flare up, often significantly. Some life stressors are inevitable, like illness, loss, volatility in relationships, financial strain, and so on. How we are impacted by stressors varies.

Stressful emotions often will trigger deleterious hormonal and epigenetic responses. Although humans are built for adaptation to stress, the type of stressors that we are exposed to in our current culture set us up for maladaptation. Our physiology is organized to help us respond appropriately with fight or flight in high-stress situations. Historically, these biological shifts were lifesaving for our ancestors as they were running into a bear in the woods or being chased across the plains by a lion. The stress response that causes pupillary dilation, increased blood pressure, decreased digestion, and adrenaline production literally enables us to mobilize or fight to preserve our lives and the lives of our loved ones.

Although the stress of an immediate threat from a predator was immense, it tended to be short lived. A few hours following the period of high stress, our ancestors' bodies would have returned to normal.

Nowadays, the pressures that cause us immense stress can last weeks, months, and years. Our bodies are not equipped to withstand chronic stress as it overtaxes our adaptation mechanisms. The results of long-term stress can be chronic high blood pressure, chronic digestive problems, like constipation, dysregulated hormones, and chronically elevated cholesterol and blood sugar.

The thing that can save us from the adverse effects of chronic stress is understanding our role in manufacturing it or relieving it. Our thoughts alone can initiate the same physiological responses as being chased by a lion or bear even if sometimes the things that are stressing us can be fairly trivial. The pressure of our responsibilities, like taking care of kids and managing a career, a marriage, and a house, as well as everyday circumstances like exposure to the news media and other people's upset and needs is, to a degree, unavoidable. We can't go live in a cave or sit on top of a rock like a hermit as a solution to the demands life puts on us. There is a way, however, to immediately, in real time, come out of our heads and gain instant healing of the effects of stress on the body and the mind. We can calm and regulate our nervous systems—reducing our stress—by bringing awareness to our hearts.

Bringing Awareness to the Heart

There is a scientific explanation for the heart's importance in creating healing and harmonious outcomes like the one I experienced while walking by the Ottawa River. According to the HeartMath Institute, the human heart has 40,000 neurons in it that are in direct communication with the brain. My five-day retreat created love-based, positive conditions in my body, which healed me.

The heart also emits the most powerful electromagnetic field of any organ in the body. In fact, the magnetic field of the heart is sixty times greater in amplitude than the electromagnetic field of the brain and 5,000 times greater in electromagnetic energy than the brain.[3]

When we change the energy in our minds, we can use it to evoke an elevated feeling in our hearts. We can then visualize this feeling being lovingly sent out from our hearts and projected into the entire universe. There's a sense, as we're doing this, that everything in and around us is shifting immediately. That healing will occur easily and naturally.

As it practically applies to healing psoriasis, the implementation of daily heart and mind rituals has the power to change our physiology and our entire bodies in present time, right in front of our eyes. These exercises are easy, pleasant, and immediately available.

The following two-minute meditation will help you regulate your emotions.

TWO-MINUTE HEART MEDITATION FOR EMOTIONAL SELF-REGULATION

Sit with your eyes closed and become aware of the presence of your heart. Begin to feel it beating and living inside of you. Place one or both hands on your chest if it helps you focus your awareness on the beating of your heart. Place your awareness on yourself as if you are someone looking down at you from above—seeing yourself *as* yourself, with your beating heart.

With your eyes closed, begin to breathe in through your nose for a count of five, hold your breath for a count of five, and breathe out for a count of five. Do this a few times in a row, settling into the pattern while feeling the sensations of your breath. Imagine that you are breathing with and from your heart, as though your heart is your entire body.

After a few cycles of breaths like this, think of someone you love, like a child or a spouse or a best friend. Thinking of my dogs sometimes helps me with this. Bring this sensation of love into your heart and allow it to affect you. See if you can use this feeling of love in your heart and the gratitude connected to it to flood your entire body, and allow that love to travel from your body as far as it will travel.

Stay with these feelings for another few breaths, and then slowly open your eyes.

You may feel tingly or warm or calm during and after this meditation—or all these things. Such feelings reflect the sort of physical and emotional shifts that will change your capacity for healing your psoriasis.

This simple meditation is incredibly powerful. I'm not asking that you believe me, I am asking only that you try it. Experiencing love and gratitude creates change for people in countless ways that aren't immediately apparent, and I am betting it will for you, too.

Participate in this practice daily and begin to observe the shifts in your mind, moods, and body.

Hebb's Law of Synaptic Connection

Even though I had long understood that my psoriasis wasn't just a skin problem, but a whole-system problem, I was surprised that modifying my thinking was the final factor necessary for healing to occur. Though I had immersed myself in understanding the quality of what I was putting into my body and my surroundings, and though I had committed myself to eating the most natural foods, taking the high-quality nutritional supplements, and using only the purest, nontoxic toiletries and household cleaning products, my skin hadn't gotten better before then. Frankly, I didn't know what else to do until the only thing left to do was the true inner work.

Since then, I have come to the conclusion that all the superfood and supplements, colonics, lotions, and potions in the world are not enough to heal psoriasis and autoimmunity in the absence of the right patterns of thought. I know it can be hard to believe, but I most emphatically encourage you to embark on a thought-noticing and thought-flipping project. Personally, I would do it in a concentrated form like I did it. Take a week. Be by yourself as much as possible, in a beautiful place, and create the space to pay attention to nothing other than your mind. Then, every time you catch a yourself thinking a thought that feels hurtful and could be damaging, flip it on the spot to a better, more self-loving, and compassionate thought. It'll probably feel tedious and forced. That's all right, just keep doing it.

In studies using high-intensity fluoroscopy microscopes and MRI imaging, neuroscientists have repeatedly demonstrated the principle of Hebb's law, first described by Donald O. Hebb, Ph.D., in 1949, that neurons will strengthen their synaptic connections when repeated thoughts (either negative or positive) occur. In other words, regardless of what the thought patterns are, the more they are repeated, the more entrenched they become as *truth* for the mind and the body.

The opposite is also true. When we discontinue a previously repeated thought pattern (like the self-deprecating thoughts I shared with you earlier, which I believe were perpetuating my autoimmunity), we actually enable for the "pruning" and weakening of those associated neuronal connections.

Whenever we replace negative, unhelpful, self-debasing language with healing, grateful, and loving language, we are literally rewiring our brains to inform our bodies differently.

The research also indicates that when a new thought occurs, new connections form between neurons (brain cells), but if these thoughts are not repeated, then those same neurons will become disconnected again.[4] Therefore, we have to be diligent in reinforcing new thinking.

Fortunately, older networks of brain cells oriented around negative thinking can be made weaker with disuse. Older thought patterns are more difficult to disrupt because the wiring has been reinforced for days, months, years, and decades. But it is possible.

For this reason, our new, more desirable thought patterns must be clear and we must very intentionally repeat them over and over until our dominant neurology has become a reflection of a new state of being.

There's something to be said about faking it until you make it—or I should say, faking it until you *become* it. Gone are the days where we separate the mind and the body.

Affirmations to Rewire the Brain

Here, I have included some examples of what affirmations may sound like. These are simply examples to lead you. You are welcome to use them verbatim, and I also encourage you to experiment with self-generated ideas that elevate your spirit. Find what works best for you.

This activity can be personalized to make it a beautiful experience. I myself like to go outside each and every morning when I first wake up, and with an open heart, as though I am speaking directly from my heart, I affirm the following ideas out loud.

- "I open my heart to the universe. I open my heart to the beauty of life."
- "Every day in every way, I am getting better and better."
- "I am beautiful and so is my skin. Thank you for this healing."
- "I love my skin and I love myself."

I also love to reflect on this piece of a traditional Navajo prayer as I walk or meditate.[5]

In beauty I walk.
With beauty before me, I walk.
With beauty behind me, I walk.
With beauty above me, I walk.
With beauty around me, I walk.
It has become beauty again.

It has become beauty again.
It has become beauty again.
It has become beauty again.

I repeat the last line, as if it were an affirmation, for as long as it feels right.

CHAPTER NINE

The Nontoxic Home and Self-Care

It's a conundrum to have psoriasis lesions on your face and want to even out the redness with makeup when you know full well that makeup reduces your skin's ability to breathe. Makeup, in and of itself, is potentially toxic and inflammation inducing.

Although the U.S. Congress has given the Food and Drug Administration (FDA) the power to regulate chemical exposure from food additives and chemicals, the personal care and cosmetic industry is expected to regulate itself as a means of addressing the risks that its products pose. Of the more than 10,000 chemicals used to formulate cosmetics, only eleven have ever been banned or restricted by the FDA as of January 2026.

Of great concern to psoriasis sufferers should be the formaldehydes, mercury, phthalates, paragons, perfluoroalkyl and polyfluoroalkyl substances (PFAS), and phenylenediamines in our personal-care products for hair and skin, which in particular irritate stressed-out and sensitive skin like ours.[1] This being said, many of us still don't want to compromise our preference for smelling nice, wearing a bit of concealer on occasion or applying a dollop of aftershave balm following a nice, close shave, and let's face it, to feeling polished and attractive. Thus, we may find ourselves pulled toward taking the risk of triggering a flareup despite knowing what we know.

Cosmetic industry labels can be very misleading. They employ catchy terms like *natural, mineral, regenerating, nutrient-filled,* and *made with organic* . . . to persuade us to feel confident about rubbing their chemicals directly on, and absorbing them through, the largest organ of our bodies—our skin.

Unfortunately, many of the organic and mineral-based makeups and skin-care products on the market that contain healthful ingredients don't work as well as the unhealthful ones. Either they look terrible or they fade or somehow "fall off" our faces within a few minutes.

Women's Makeup

There are a couple of makeup alternatives that I have grown to trust. Two of my personal favorite cosmetic collections are:

- **Jane Iredale.** Mineral-based, natural-ingredient makeup that is as beautiful as it is nontoxic. I love their concealer, lip gloss, lipstick, and eye shadow.

Jane Iredale is the real deal. Established over twenty-five years ago, the company made one of the first true mineral makeups, which is long lasting but light.

- **Jones Road.** A moisturizing makeup that I use for everyday cheek and lip color. The makeup is beautiful and moisturizing. I like that Jones Road has made a commitment to hold itself to an even higher standard than the European Union standard for makeup (which is better than the American and Canadian standards). Their cosmetics are free of all the toxins of great concern listed above.

Men's Shaving Products

Of course, women are not the only ones who need to be concerned about toxic self-care products. Men need to be concerned with products that touch their skin, like the shaving products they use daily.[2]

Many of the common ingredients found in shaving creams and gels include side effects and warnings specific to inflammatory skin reactions like dermatitis, and skin irritation allergic reactions. Look for shaving products that are free of fragrance, parabens, sodium laureth sulfate (SLES), propylene and butylene glycols, and triethanolamine.[3]

Hair Coloring

I started coloring my hair when I was in my mid-thirties. I started noticing the occasional gray hair on my head in my early thirties, so by the time I was in my early forties I was coloring my hair every three weeks. I wanted to avoid gray roots "breaking through." Being particular about my appearance, the idea of presenting myself with a "skunk stripe" made me crazy.

Back then, I was coloring my hair myself so that I could make use of supposedly organic hair coloring. Even so, what I noticed was that with every application of hair coloring my scalp would burn and I would get an angry, red, stripe-like spot (looking like psoriasis) between my eyebrows for hours, and sometimes days, after application. As time went by, I also began to notice that I would feel a bit nauseous and fatigued on "hair-coloring days."

Eventually, despite my numerous attempts to ignore all of the signals my body was displaying that the products I was using were toxic and my body was unable to stand up successfully to being poisoned, I had to get real with myself and make the difficult decision to stop coloring my hair. For two years, I found myself standing in front of the mirror having pep talks with myself as my gray hair was exposed. I had to shed the false premise that my new appearance had me looking like a witch, old, and bedraggled. As a woman, this was one of the most difficult things I've ever done.

It's embarrassing to admit that I gave so much head space to the issue of growing out my gray because I realize that the privilege of such vanity is very much a first-world problem. Now, being over three years into this *au naturel* look, I'm actually feeling more empowered. In fact, I might even go as far as saying that I might be rocking the sexy silver look!

A simple Google search for "hair coloring and psoriasis" brought me results on "how to do it safely" and "how to color if you have scalp psoriasis." However, further searching revealed numerous papers written about hair color being a "risk for autoimmunity." The chemical p-paraphenylendiamine (PPD) found in hair colorings is meant to darken the hair. But it's also used in dyeing furs and textiles that may come into contact with our skin.

With psoriasis, we're looking at the toxic insult of PPD in two parts because any irritant placed on psoriatic skin can cause exacerbations by means of contact and absorption. The skin, being the largest organ in the body, will absorb chemical toxins directly into the body in a manner that is analogous to ingesting or injecting a toxin. Remember that the skin is not a barrier; it is more of a porous mesh that relays information to the rest of the body as a first line of interpretation and defense.

Breathing toxic gases output by products, such as these, is another way these toxins harm us.

According to the EPA, PPD can cause inflammatory skin conditions (eczematoid dermatitis) along with organ toxicity—and even organ failure. According to the research, skin reactions to PPD can be found from the contact point and with individuals who have no "on-contact" symptoms.[4]

Being that most women and some men spend some time of their lives coloring their hair, the conversation of hair coloring and the perpetuation of toxicity becomes unavoidable. This is an elephant in the room which has taken up a lot of space.

Over the few years that I, myself, ignored the elephant by using supposedly natural hair coloring, including some organic brands I picked up at health-food stores and was provided at an Aveda salon. Ultimately, I came to the conclusion that there is no such thing as an entirely safe permanent hair color. Permanent hair color formulations require alkaline agents to open the hair shaft before introducing dyes. Toxins of this sort include diaminophenoxyethanol, hydrochloride, polysorbate, ammonium hydroxide, toluene, and sulfate, all of which can cause significant issues, including severe skin reactions.[5]

Tattoos

Tattoos have been around for over 6,000 years, dating back to ancient Egypt. I love the idea and personal expression of tattoos. They can individualize our creativity, and even our spirituality, but unlike 6,000 years ago, when people used organic compounds in their inks, today, tattoo ink is hazardous for those of us with psoriasis.

In the fall of 2024, I got a simple, dainty, feminine-looking tattoo. This black tattoo, located on my inner arm, is smaller than the palm of my hand. Not long after I got inked, I noticed a small plaque of psoriasis directly on the tattoo–the first blemish I'd had in many years. Initially, I assumed that it occurred because of skin irritation caused by the tattoo needle. A few months later, however, I noticed that I had seven or so more additional small plaques on my lower back and upper abdomen. Apparently something more was going on.

I don't know why it had never occurred to me that tattoo ink could be toxic. When I did some research, I learned that it is high in metals and metalloids: chromium, lead, arsenic, mercury, nickel, and copper. Red inks may contain the most damaging levels of chromium, iron oxide, and cadmium, placing them in the category of "most toxic."[6]

The commonly used carbon black inks contain polycyclic aromatic hydrocarbons, which are known to exacerbate autoimmune disease and allergic reactions.[7]

The inks used in tattoos aren't assessed by the FDA or by any other safety regulation agency in the United States. Out of seventy-three tattoo inks available in Sweden, 93 percent of the tattoo ink samples bought and tested did not follow the labeling rules for trace metals as set by European laws, and 61 percent the inks had harmful red pigments.[8]

Tattoo ink isn't pervasive in the blood stream, but it does appear to accumulate in the lymphatic system and in the liver. If you are concerned about the potential toxicity of any of your tattoos, then chelation and cellular detoxification protocols may be appropriate. In order to chelate, seek the help of a naturopathic physician or a functional medicine doctor well-versed in chelation.

Household Cleaning Products

Most traditional cleaning products are made with phosphate compounds and other skin- and lung-irritating chemicals. Chemicals like sodium dodecylbenzene sulfonate (SDBS), a widely used surfactant (a surface-acting agent used to dissolve grime and grease), which are absorbed through the skin, are known to cause and skin and liver damage.[9]

To keep chemical stressors out of our homes, it is necessary to use cleaning products that are free of synthetic (petroleum-derived) surfactants and detergents. Being that we have plenty of chemical exposure everywhere else, being in control of our cleaning products, ideally using only natural ones formulated with plant-based surfactants and biodegradable Castille soaps; olive, hemp, and coconut oils; essential oils; and vinegar is a great place to start.

There are ways to make your own nontoxic, natural products. I recommend the recipes in the book *The*

Naturally Clean Home by Karyn Siegel-Maier. If you would prefer to purchase cleaning products, try brands like Seventh Generation, Ecos, Common Ground, Dr. Bronner's, Blueland, Biokleen, and Bon Ami. These companies are dedicated to creating nontoxic, natural, and often organic, products that won't cause toxic stress in our bodies in the name of cleaning.

Watch out for your dish soap and dishwasher soap for the obvious reason that, on a daily basis, you are literally eating their chemical residue. Some dishwasher soaps include formaldehyde-releasing agents as well as synthetic fragrances and surfactants.

Included in the red flags of concern are products that contain polyethylene glycol (PEG). This chemical, which is commonly found in dish soap, can trigger autoimmune responses. PEG is found in dishwasher pods and cleaning products like Mr. Clean, Cascade, Jet Dry, and Finish as well. It can also be found in Ajax and Murphy Oil Soap. Be cautious even of brands labeled as "natural" and "organic."[10]

It should be noted that the Pfizer/BioNTech Covid-19 vaccine contains PEG and that sensitivity to PEG is a documented contraindication to receiving this particular vaccine. This may explain the Covid-19 vaccine link to increased susceptibility to the onset and exacerbation of psoriasis.[11]

Phthalates are cautioned against as well. Phthalates, found in dish soap, air freshener, laundry detergent, carpet deodorizer, dusting spray, and other household cleaning products, have been linked to alterations in immune system function, including overactivity of the immune system and autoimmunity. Be on alert for their possible presence when reading ingredient labels, because phthalates are often included under the ingredient "perfume" or "fragrance."[12] Specific brands to avoid include Glade, Oust, and Simple Green, but there are many others.

PART THREE

THE 90-DAY, PSORIASIS-HEALING PROGRAM

CHAPTER TEN

Three Months to Better Skin

In this chapter, I will lay out an exact protocol to follow to heal your psoriasis over the course of the next ninety days. This protocol has been meticulously designed and redesigned multiple times over and tested on the patients in my practice. I have done my best to make the instructions as simple and straightforward as possible. Here's an overview.

During the 90-Day Psoriasis-Healing Program, you will be adhering to specific guidelines for:

- Diet.
- Supplementation.
- Lifestyle modification.
- Mindset shift.

The dietary protocol you will use during the first five days of the protocol (and optionally for the first five days of Months 2 and 3) is the most stringent because these days are the intervals when healing is being kickstarted. The purpose of the diet you eat on Days 1–5 (of every thirty) is to detox and rejuvenate. You also need to take the pressure off your elimination system while your body is cleansing, so you want to introduce only the nutrients that will assist your body in doing this fundamental healing work. This precise protocol resembles fasting (though you still get to eat), and is called the Five-Day Fasting-Mimicking Cleanse.

On Days 6–30, you will eat cleanly according to the guidance of the well-known autoimmune protocol (AIP) diet. This protocol, whose intent is to reduce chronic inflammation, is the gold standard for healing autoimmune conditions like psoriasis in my opinion.

Although the dietary protocols you follow over this ninety-day stretch of time may seem tedious, they should be followed diligently. At the end, it is my belief that you will be glad you did.

What has been helpful for me when I am feeling challenged while implementing temporary food restrictions like these is to rely on affirmations. I remind myself, “Everything is temporary” and “Every day in every way I am getting better and better.”

Do your best to stay strong and have some compassion for yourself.

Let’s begin with instructions for the five-day fasting-mimicking cleanse. The “big idea” here is to give your body a chance to heal itself.

Dietary Guidelines Days 1–5: The Fasting-Mimicking Cleanse

Fasting (usually defined as forswearing food and beverages, except water, for a specified period) has been shown to effectively reduce inflammation, aid with cellular cleanup, and boost cellular rejuvenation. Studies of the effects of fasting have demonstrated a healing effect with autoimmunity, chronic inflammation, cancer, weight loss, blood sugar levels, heart disease, lipid profiles, and neurological inflammatory processes. However, I do not advise you to restrict *all* food and beverages. Instead I advocate this fasting-mimicking regimen that tricks the body into thinking you are fasting and proves similar results. Adherence of this sort is much easier.

The Five-Day Fasting-Mimicking Cleanse, whose purpose for people with psoriasis is to kick-start the healing process, as outlined in the following pages, should be followed for the first five days of the month and optionally repeated once per month for two months of the program. This cleanse is based on the research of biochemist and longevity researcher Valter Longo, Ph.D., a leading researcher on fasting. All of Dr. Longo's published research is based on studies in which participants underwent three fasting-mimicking cycles.

I have guided 200 people through the same variation of the Fasting-Mimicking Cleanse as is described in this book. Over 165 of them got at least 90 percent better while the rest saw some significant improvement.

The fasting-mimicking cleanse you are being invited to do to heal your psoriasis has been shown to rapidly decrease inflammation, reduce symptoms of autoimmunity, and aid with overall healing of plaques and skin lesions. A lot will be going on at the cellular level, including detoxification and regeneration.

The cleanse is calorie-restricted, with the consumption of 1,100 calories on Day 1 and 750 calories per day on Days 2–5. It is also protein restricted. During this fasting-mimicking period, the ratio of macronutrients in your meals will be 47 percent carbohydrates, 45 percent fats, and only 8 percent proteins. The cleanse is sugar free, dairy free, and meat free, and on Days 2–5, legume free and grain free.

In years past, because of desiring to cleanse my body of toxins, I attempted both water fasting and broth fasting. Neither was satisfactory. I found that, due to my busy schedule, it was very difficult to dive into either kind of liquid fasting without feeling very depleted and nonfunctional. This five-day dietary regimen tricks the body into behaving as if you are fasting, but without the uncomfortable effects of complete calorie restriction.

We begin the protocol with a fasting-mimicking cleanse as a reset to the inflammation-driven, rapid turnover of skin cells that defines psoriasis. When performed for the first five days of the month in tandem with supplementation and lifestyle modifications, it creates a pattern of disruption to the chronicity of the inflammatory culprit that is psoriasis. Based on a self-assessment of how well you are healing, you have the option to repeat the cleanse at the beginning of Months 2 and 3.

If you have never participated in a cleanse before, your first experience of eliminating familiar foods from your diet may feel challenging. Please do remember, however, that the cleanse lasts only five days, and any hunger pangs or cravings you may feel are normal. Although hunger can cause us to feel panicky, there is no real danger of starvation during this interval. Although fasting-mimicking takes commitment, it can be worth it.

WARNING: *The Five-Day Fasting-Mimicking Cleanse is not appropriate for pregnant or nursing mothers. Nor is it appropriate for anyone who is underweight. Anyone eighty years old or older or sixteen years old or younger should not do this cleanse.*

The Five-Day Fasting-Mimicking Cleanse is also not appropriate for those taking blood sugar-lowering drugs or weight-loss medications. Please consult with your doctor about the safest way to temporarily discontinue these drugs for the purpose of participating in this cleanse and to assess whether or not the cleanse is appropriate for your personal situation.

The Five-Day Fasting-Mimicking Cleanse Menu

The following menu is a specific guide that in its totality incorporates the ideal ratio of carbs, fats, and proteins you need. I hope you enjoy the recipes. Following the completion of the cleanse, the recipes in this menu can be incorporated into your repertoire of meals by adding meats, sprouted grains, and other Eat This Food List ingredients to them (*see* Chapter 11 for recipes).

Caloric intake	Breakfast	Lunch	Dinner
Day 1 — 1,100 calories	Oatmeal	Hummus and Sweet Potato Platter w/ Cabbage Salad	Ginger Carrot Soup
Day 2 — 750 calories	Mixed Berry Fruit Salad with Pine Nuts	Avocado Shakshuka	Paleo Pad Thai

Day 3 — 750 calories	Chia Seed Pudding	Beets Fricassee	Potatoes & Veggies w/Kale Pesto
Day 4 — 750 calories	Lemon, Kiwi, and Strawberry Smoothie	Mushroom Soup	Veggie Hash w/ Leeks, Cauli-flower, & Asparagus
Day 5 — 750 Calories	Pineapple Kale Smoothie	Apple, Almond, & Arugula Salad	Broccoli Cream Soup

Dietary Guidelines Days 6–30: The Autoimmune Protocol Diet

For now, I recommend that you entirely avoid:

- Eggs and products that include eggs.
- Dairy (milk, cream, butter, whipped cream, cream cheese, cottage cheese, cheese).

- All grains (wheat, barley, quinoa, spelt, rye, rice, millet).
- All legumes (kidney beans, black beans, garbanzo beans/chickpeas, navy beans, pinto beans, lentils, peas, and any products made from them).
- All sugars (white sugar, brown sugar, confectioner's sugar, corn syrup, and molasses/treacle) and products that contain added sugars, including fructose).
- Coffee.
- Alcoholic beverages.
- Nuts and seeds (peanuts, almonds, cashews, walnuts, pecans, hazelnuts, Brazil nuts; and chia seeds, flax seeds, sunflower seeds, and so on).
- All produce in the nightshades family (eggplants, tomatoes, tomatillos, potatoes, cayenne pepper, chili pepper, and Bell peppers).
- Soybeans (edamame) and products made from soy.

What you should eat is high-quality protein, vegetables, and fruits not on the list above, coconut products, like coconut yogurts and baked goods made with alternate flours like cassava. There are many AIP recipe websites with great guidance and ideas to help create a satisfactory menu. Please note that the AIP portion of this ninety-day fasting-mimicking diet is not intended to be calorie restricted. It's important to ensure that you receive adequate calorie intake.

Although quite strict, the Program will establish a new foundation of health with which to build upon. It should be duly noted that many of the foods eliminated while on the AIP diet are not "harmful foods" or foods which should come with a sense of guilt or negativity once reintroduced. This is an important point because again, the way we communicate with ourselves is important and "guilty thoughts" over foods sets a physiological stage which can result in the opposite of a healing outcome. These foods are simply being temporarily eliminated in order to give the gut and the body a "break" and to make space for the return to a healthy state.

Supplementation Guidelines

The second element of the Psoriasis-Healing Program is supplementation. For ninety days, including the five days of cleansing at the beginning of each thirty-day cycle, I recommend taking the following twelve supplements. For specific brand recommendations, please visit my website: AnikStMartin.com/skinonfire.

1. A multivitamin incorporating trace minerals (including magnesium and zinc).

   Recommended dose: As per product recommendation.

2. Omega 3 fatty acids. Studies show that when the EPA and DHA fatty acids found in fish are used together, they can help reduce inflammation in as little as four weeks.[1] *Recommended dose:* 2,000

milligrams per day, split between morning and evening.

If you are a vegetarian or vegan, please visit my website for the names of algae- or flax-based omega-3 fatty acid supplements.

Incorporating fatty fish, like wild-caught salmon and sardines canned in extra-virgin olive oil in your diet is also highly recommended.

WARNING: *Many fish oil supplements are tainted with toxins like mercury, and the oils are prone to rancidity. Please be cautious about the brands you choose and store your omega 3 supplements in the refrigerator.*

3. Glutathione. This antioxidant has been shown to be deficient in those with psoriasis, and supplementation with it has been shown to help relieve psoriasis symptoms.[2] The most absorbable kind is liposomal glutathione.

   Recommended dose: 2,000 milligrams per day.

4. Resveratrol. Found in the gingko biloba plant, the flavonoid resveratrol has powerful anti-inflammatory and healing properties and has been shown to help clear up psoriasis.[3] It is naturally found in foods like red wine, red grapes, dark chocolate, and pomegranate, but for the ninety-day protocol, I recommend resveratrol in supplement form. Please note that some resveratrol is combined with

quercetin—which is optimal, saving you the trouble of obtaining a separate quercetin (see #5 below). See my website for a link.

Recommended dose: 400 milligrams per day.

5. Quercetin. Derived from fruits and vegetables, the natural polyphenolic flavonoid quercetin has significant antioxidant and anti-inflammatory effects and has been demonstrated to be of significant help in healing psoriatic lesions.[4]

   Recommended dose: 400 milligrams per day.

6. Vitamin B complex that includes a methylated folate (vitamin B9). Take to improve your methylation and generally detox.

   Recommended dose: 1 capsule per day, or 400–600 micrograms.

7. Turmeric/curcumin. Curcumin is the active ingredient in turmeric that makes it a powerful anti-inflammatory. You can also get curcumin by eating foods with turmeric, like yellow curry.

   Recommended dose: 1,000 milligrams per day.

8. Choline. Choline supplements may help reduce the severity of psoriasis by modulating inflammatory cytokines and thereby improving cellular health. *Recommended dose:* 1,000 milligrams per day.

9. GI Tract Repair, which typically comes as a powder. The ideal gut-healing supplement is made up of L-glutamine powder, colostrum, N-acetyl

glucosamine, slippery elm bark powder, MSM, Rutin NF, and aloe vera leaf.

Recommended dose: One scoop per day.

WARNING: *Some products of this type contain shellfish (lobster, crab, and/or shrimp) and milk.*

See my website for the names of products that do not contain shellfish or dairy.

10. Vitamin D in combination with vitamin K. *Recommended dose:* 8,000 IUs per day.
11. Probiotics. Necessary to restore and maintain the integrity of the microbiome.

    Recommended dose: Maximum recommended amount as per package insert.
12. Green Vibrance by Vibrant Health®. This is a plant-based green superfood powder.
    Recommended dose: 1 scoop per day.

I am aware that this may seem like quite a bit. Please remember, you are kickstarting healing, detoxification, and anti-inflammatory processes in your body. These supplements should be considered essential for the program.

With the assumption that your body's healing is well underway following the ninety-day program, the intensity of supplementation can lessen on the first day of Week 13.

I find that because my days are busy and sometimes unpredictable, taking my supplements in the morning to ensure that I actually do take them is the best plan for me. If you are a more organized person than me, a daily schedule might look like the supplementation menu on the next page.

Supplementation Menu

Morning	Midday	Evening
Multivitamin and trace mineral	Resveratrol	Choline
Omega 3 fatty acid	Glutathione	Vitamin D
Probiotic	Probiotic	Probiotic
Curcumin	B Complex	Curcumin
Green Vibrance		Quercetin
GI Repair	GI Repair	GI Repair

Days 1–30 Lifestyle Modifications

Soothe and Restore Your Nervous System

While you're undergoing nutritional detoxification and healing over the course of these ninety days, it is important to simultaneously soothe and restore the balance of your nervous system. Rest should be a priority. Do your best to keep your level of emotional stress low and focus on seven to ten hours of uninterrupted sleep per night. This period is an excellent time to practice the healing techniques you learned in Chapter 8, such as the Two-Minute Heart Meditation for Emotional Self-Regulation and positive affirmations.

As an accompaniment to the nutrition and supplementation recommendations I've given you, additional lifestyle recommendation are chiropractic care, forgiveness, and sleep to soothe your central nervous system.

CHIROPRACTIC CARE

Having been a doctor of chiropractic for over two decades, during which time I've cared for thousands of adults, including pregnant women, and children. I have observed, first hand, the potential for healing that can be brought forth through the removal of interference on the nervous system.

If chiropractic care seems like an odd addition to the 90-Day Psoriasis-Healing Program, I would ask you to reconsider what you've come to know. The brain, as you know, connects to and sends all of its energy to the body through the spinal cord, which is housed in and protected by the spine. When spinal segments become displaced (a condition known as *subluxation)* due to physical, chemical, and emotional injury and stress, this interferes with the nervous system's potential for integrating information and energy from different organs, cells, and tissues. When spinal subluxation goes unchecked, entire sections of the spine can become distorted and affected; and when the spine becomes distorted, organ systems will degenerate and become sick over time, thereby dampening our ability to heal.

Due to the fact that psoriasis is autoimmune in nature, an optimally functioning spine and nervous system are an absolute necessity. Studies have shown that chiropractic care helps the body adapt to stress through the balancing of cortisol, the stress hormone produced by the adrenal glands.[5] Chiropractic care improves the function of the brain at the frontal cortex, situated just behind the forehead, which is responsible for cognition, problem solving, fine motor skills, and impulse control.[6]

Research has also shown that a chiropractic adjustment improves the conduction potential of energy from the brain to the rest of the body.[7] If we can agree that healing is largely dependent on energy, then a lifestyle approach that is energy driven is necessary. In fact, postural correction enables us to have more longevity. When we correct the positioning of these bones so the nerves and fluids in them are not impinged, we literally live longer.[8]

Additional studies have shown that chiropractic care makes us more self-aware.[9] In other words, when a person receives a chiropractic adjustment, they enhance the level of energy with which they adapt and heal and connect to their environment.

During the 90-Day Healing Psoriasis Program, I would recommend seeing a chiropractor three times per week to promote nervous system healing and to support detoxification. Be sure to explain what you are trying to achieve to the doctor and make a plan that applies to your specific condition.

NOTE: Please seek out a qualified and licensed doctor of chiropractic for specific recommendations.

The recommended frequency of care, once your nervous system has returned to a healing state, is once per week, as a lifestyle habit. Tending to the nervous system on a weekly basis allows us to adapt to the world around us better, and it allows us to interpret and process all of life's stressors in a resilient manner, instead of swimming against the current through the impact which stressors have on our nervous systems.

IF YOU'VE EXPERIENCED A TRAUMA, DO YOUR BEST TO FORGIVE

There have been many books and scientific studies published demonstrating the often overlooked, but absolutely essential importance of not staying stuck in deleterious thinking associated with past trauma. Those of us who know the thing that "happened to us" — perhaps because there was a clear "before" and "after" to the onset of our psoriasis—are both gifted and cursed by the knowledge. If we find ourselves swimming in an ocean of resentment for perceived and/or actual injustices, it does us no good. The neurochemical cocktail served to us by negative emotions that come with viewing ourselves as victims is not of service to our healing.

Forgiveness helps us take responsibility for where we are today health-wise, even if certain decisions that led to our psoriasis were made on our behalf and were beyond our control—like they were for me as a child. Forgive your parents. Forgive your body. Forgive your choices. Forgive your doctors. Forgive anyone for whom you have a lingering resentment. Forgive yourself and let it go.

SLEEP

Ninety percent of psoriasis sufferers report being sleep deprived due to overall difficulty with sleep. There appears to be a vicious cycle in operation here. The discomfort associated with psoriasis, including itching and burning and emotional upset, can cause insomnia.

Then, by inhibiting healing, sleep deprivation promotes the inflammatory state. Although there has been no conclusion as to whether sleep deprivation comes as a result of psoriasis or contributes to the psoriasis, we do know that loss of sleep and psoriasis are often connected.[10]

Our bodies heal while we sleep and the better we sleep, the more accessible healing becomes. The old adage "Early to bed, early to rise, makes a man healthy, wealthy and wise" should be taken as advice. Adopting an early bedtime as a lifestyle is the best way to ensure that you get seven to ten hours per night while you are healing. Remember that without enough sleep, the body can't heal *even* if we're doing everything else we are supposed to do.

Three More Game-Changing Habits

I consider the follow three health habits *game-changers* because they have no adverse effects. These habits make me feel so good that they have been extended into every aspect of my life—thereby having an effect not just on my skin but also on how I show up in the world.

These habits are powerful because they help us with everything from digestion and immune system resilience to sleep, detoxification, and overall adaptation.

In order, the habits I recommend you embrace are:

- Adequate hydration.
- Drinking sole water.
- Taking saunas.

If these methods are new to you or you are skeptical about their potential contribution to healing psoriasis, please do your best to keep an open mind. Willingness to experiment is the key to being successful for ninety days.

ADEQUATE HYDRATION

During this ninety-day period of accelerated detoxification and healing, I recommend that you drink a minimum of half your body weight in ounces of water each day. (Example: Someone who weighs 150 pounds requires a minimum of 75 ounces of water daily).

People with psoriasis potentially may develop restless leg syndrome, a neurological condition that causes a very strong urge to move the legs and may be accompanied by sensations of itching, burning or skin crawling which improve when the limb is moved. In my experience, restless leg syndrome often comes as result of mineral and electrolyte depletion, along with dehydration. These depletions also are a direct cause of sleep problems and insomnia.

In order to combat depletion and dehydration, water intake is important, along with the daily replenishment of electrolytes and minerals. I've worked with hundreds of patients over the years who've handled their restless leg syndromes successfully simply with hydration.

DRINKING SOLE WATER

For decades now, we've been taught that salt is harmful to our health, and so it should be greatly minimized, if not avoided. This may be true in the case of salt in high-sodium processed food, such as canned soup. A small can of soup typically contains over 1,200 milligrams of sodium. Highly refined table salt, which typically lacks trace minerals that would be beneficial to us, also should be restricted. According to the American Heart Association (AHA), we should consume no more than 3,300 milligrams of sodium per day, and ideally no more than 1,500 milligrams for a healthy adult.[11]

For ages now, however, people have been consuming high-quality salts that nature has laced with trace minerals to enrich our health and address various health concerns. Because sodium chloride (salt) is essential to vital functions in our bodies, such as controlling our fluid balance, conducting nerve impulses, and contracting and relaxing our muscles, adding high-quality salt to our food is highly recommended.

The daily habit of drinking a small amount of homemade salt water, known as *sole,* can help with constipation, heart rate regulation, blood sugar balancing, and sleep. For the important purpose, during these twelve weeks of intentionally healing our psoriasis, sole aids detoxification and improves digestion and bowel elimination. Thus it will specifically help to decrease skin inflammation. For those of us who are histamine reactive, sole is also known to aid in the body's production of antihistamine enzymes that degrade histamine.[12]

Sole has all of these benefits because it balances the positively and negatively charged ions in the body by allowing essential substances to better enter and exit the cell walls.

HOW TO MAKE SOLE

The salt crystals which are traditionally used to make sole water are harvested from the salt mines in the Himalayan Mountains of Pakistan. (*See* Resources for recommended crystals.)

Ingredients

2 cups Himalayan salt crystals
4 cups filtered water

Instructions

Fill a mason jar to the halfway marks with Himalayan salt, and top with filtered water. Place on a sunny window sill for twenty-four to forty-eight hours. Although the sun isn't necessary for the crystals to dissolve, those who have studied sole believe that sunlight activates the eighty-four trace minerals held within the Himalayan salt, thereby activating the energetic and healing properties.

Every morning, before ingesting anything else, including coffee, drink a large glass of lukewarm filtered water to which you've added a splash of sole. This beverage should taste slightly salty—palpably, but enjoyably so, rather than strongly salty like the ocean.

When sole becomes familiar to you, you will notice how the concentration of sole you require on a daily basis changes according to your body's needs. Some mornings you may need to dilute the water for it to seem palatable. Some mornings, you won't be able to taste the salt at all and may need to add another splash.

Drinking sole on a daily basis can be life changing if making it a habit improves the quality of your digestion, sleep, and overall health.

SAUNAS

Bathing in heat, as a ritual and for cleansing, purification and healing has been used for thousands of years across multiple cultures. Although there are no studies which look at psoriasis and sauna use specifically, many people anecdotally report that regular sauna use helps reduce skin inflammation and other psoriasis symptoms.

A comprehensive study published in 2021 looking at 2,300 sauna users in Finland, showed the tremendous advantage of regular sauna use on cardiovascular health, respiratory function, longevity, mental health, lipid profiles, immune function, and chronic inflammation.

Heat adaptation and sweating facilitate higher excretion of some heavy metals including aluminum (3.75-fold), cadmium (twenty-five-fold), cobalt (seven-fold), and lead (seventeen-fold). Knowing that cadmium toxicity has been linked to psoriasis and that those with psoriasis tend to have greater difficulty with DNA methylation which aids in heavy metal detoxing, it stands to reason that "sweating it out" may be very beneficial.

One of the body's protective responses to heat exposure is through the production of heat shock proteins. These proteins aid with cellular healing, immune function, and cell cycle regulation, and they help protect against cellular stress thereby being protective against chronic disease.

Saunas and heat exposure also help promote the production of specific interleukin 10 which is an "anti-inflammation" cytokine. The study also demonstrated a decreased and better balance of C-reactive protein which is a blood marker of chronic inflammation.

The above referenced study was conducted using dry saunas which are saunas whereby water can be poured onto the heating element's hot rocks to create moisture (as opposed to a steam bath). The beneficial effects appear to come from the body's production of heat and through the detox effect connected to sweating.

The study does compare sauna use of once per week versus four to seven times per week and finds a significantly higher overall benefit with the latter. Having a home sauna feels like a dream come true, I use mine almost daily, but prior to obtaining one for home use, I would frequent my local YMCA which boasts a Finnish dry sauna. I strongly encourage you to seek out a membership in a gym with a sauna to see if the benefits of a sauna to you would warrant building a home unit. (See Resources for sauna supply recommendations).[13]

What to Do After the Psoriasis-Healing Program Ends

For some people, the Psoriasis-Healing Program will be enough to completely heal their skin. One to three rounds of the fasting-mimicking cleanse and dietary change plus supplementation along with lifestyle modifications has done wonders for me and my chiropractic patients. The AIP diet in particular has been documented to decrease autoimmunity markers and inflammatory markers in the bloodstream, so you can expect it to stabilize your health.

DIETARY GUIDANCE

If your symptoms have abated, eat according to the guidelines in Chapters 6 and 7.

If you are experiencing a more deeply ingrained state of inflammation, you may still require additional gut and autoimmunity healing. After the initial twelve weeks, you should carry on with the AIP diet for another three months, but move on to the new supplement guidelines described below.

Supplementation for Stabilizing Your Health

With the assumption that healing will be well underway for you by Week 12, the intensity of supplementation lessens starting in Week 13. Now, I want you to take:

1. Multivitamin and trace minerals (including magnesium). *Dose:* 1 tablet per day, per instructions on the bottle.
2. Omega-3 fatty acid. *Dose:* 2,000 milligrams per day.
3. Probiotic. *Dose:* maximum recommended on your product of choice.
4. GI Repair. *Dose:* 1 scoop per day for an additional nine months.
5. Vitamin D. *Dose:* 2,000 IUs per day.
6. Methylated B-complex. *Dose:* 1 capsule per day.
7. Green Vibrance. *Dose:* 1 scoop per day.

CHAPTER ELEVEN

Fasting-Mimicking Cleanse Recipes

Please note that all recipes presented here will produce two servings. If you are participating in the cleanse by yourself, please halve the recipes or freeze the second half and save for a later cleanse.

Fasting-Mimicking Breakfasts

OATMEAL

Ingredients

1 cup rolled oats
1 cup water
1 ounce walnuts
1 cup raspberries or blueberries
16 ounces unsweetened coconut milk (from a refrigerated carton—not canned)

Instructions

Cook the oats in the water, over medium heat (5–10 minutes to get creamy).

Add nuts, berries, and coconut milk and serve.

TIP: Two small (about 4-ounce) apples may substitute for berries.

MIXED BERRY SALAD WITH PINE NUTS

Ingredients

2 cups mixed berries (strawberries, raspberries, blackberries)

Juice of 2 lemons

1 tablespoon pine nuts

Instructions

Cut the stems from the berries, rinse, then slice into bite-sized pieces.

Squeeze lemon juice over the fruit and sprinkle on pine nuts.

CHIA SEED PUDDING

This recipe must be prepared the night before. Please note that although it is recommended to avoid seeds and nuts for the remainder of the ninety days, seeds are included in the five-day cleanse in order to reach an 8 percent protein macro.

Ingredients

¾ cup unsweetened coconut milk (from a refrigerated carton—not canned)
⅓ cup chia seeds
½ teaspoon vanilla extract
¾ teaspoon honey (omit if you are a vegan)
⅔ cup blueberries, fresh or frozen

Instructions

Blend all ingredients except the chia seeds in a blender until smooth.

Pour the blended mixture into a bowl, and whisk in the chia seeds.

Portion the mixture into two small glass jars or a large glass container and place in the refrigerator for at least four hours, or overnight, to allow it to gel.

Serve in the glass or in bowls. Enjoy.

LEMON, KIWI, AND STRAWBERRY SMOOTHIE

Ingredients

7 strawberries
1 banana
1 kiwi
Juice of 1 lemon
½ cup water, cold
Ice (optional)

Instructions

Cut the strawberries, banana, and kiwi into pieces and place them in a blender. Add the lemon juice and water, and blend for about 30 seconds. Serve immediately.

TIP: I like to add quite a bit of ice to thicken it up and it seems to taste so much better when it's very cold. If you freeze cut-up banana pieces ahead of time, you won't need ice.

PINEAPPLE KALE SMOOTHIE

Ingredients

3 cups loosely packed kale (or spinach), stems removed
1½ heaping cups frozen pineapple chunks
1½ large, frozen, ripe bananas, cut into chunks
1½ cups unsweetened coconut milk (from a refrigerated carton—not canned)
½ tablespoon chia seeds
½-inch piece fresh, peeled ginger (optional)
1 cup ice

Instructions

In a large, high-speed blender, add in all the ingredients and blend on high for 1–2 minutes, or until all ingredients are well combined. If necessary to thin the smoothie, add in more milk and blend again.

Fasting-Mimicking Lunches

HUMMUS AND SWEET POTATO PLATTER WITH CABBAGE SALAD

Everything can be prepared ahead of time and assembled on a platter just prior to serving.

Ingredients for the Hummus

1 cup chickpeas, drained and rinsed
1 teaspoon tahini
2 teaspoons extra-virgin olive oil
1 tablespoon lemon juice
Pinch of salt
Water (optional)

Ingredients for the Platter

1 small sweet potato, prebaked in the oven (see note*)
2 cups cabbage
Pinch of salt
1 tablespoon olive oil
2 teaspoons apple cider vinegar
Pinch of black pepper
2 raw carrots, peeled and chopped into two-bite-long sticks
1 cup bite-sized pieces of cauliflower florets
1 cup shredded green lettuce or arugula

Instructions for the Hummus
Combine the chickpeas, tahini, extra-virgin olive oil, lemon juice, and salt in a blender or food processor until it reaches the consistency you prefer.

Add water to the hummus, one teaspoon at a time, if it feels too thick.

TIP: Adding a few cubes of ice to the blender makes extra-fluffy hummus.

Preparing the Salad Platter
Warm the precooked sweet potato (preferable) in the oven at 325 degrees for 10–15 minutes or cook it now.

Shred the cabbage with a cheese shredder, massage with the salt, olive oil, apple cider vinegar, and pepper. Mix the lettuce (or arugula) into it.

Serve the sweet potato with the raw carrot sticks and cauliflower florets over the salad. The hummus can be used as a dipping sauce or as a dressing, whichever you prefer.

TIP: You can remove the sweet potato and add more hummus if you like, but no more than a half cup of hummus per serving.

**NOTE:* It is recommended that you cook the sweet potato at 350 degrees in the oven until tender (approximately 30–35 minutes) the day prior and refrigerate it until you're ready to prepare the dish. Precooking followed by overnight refrigeration reduces the glycemic index value (sugar spike) of the sweet potato.

AVOCADO SHAKSHUKA

Ingredients

¼ teaspoon cumin seeds
1¼ tablespoons extra-virgin olive oil
⅓ cup onion, diced
1 large Bell pepper
¼ cup parsley
2 tablespoons cilantro
1⅓ cups tomatoes
Pinch of cayenne pepper
Pinch of black pepper
1 bay leaf
A few tablespoons of water
¾ cup avocado, sliced

Instructions

Roast the cumin seeds in a pan over low heat without oil (dry), until fragrant.

Add the olive oil and onions to the pan and sauté for 5 minutes, until translucent.

Cut the Bell peppers into thin, bite-sized strips and season with the parsley and cilantro. Add to the onions and sauté for another 10 minutes, stirring occasionally.

Cut tomatoes into small pieces and season with cayenne and black pepper. Then, add to pan along with the bay leaf. Cook in the pan at a low temperature for 15 minutes, adding small amounts of water occasionally to get a light saucy consistency.

Remove bay leaf.

Serve on two plates and add sliced avocado on top of the shakshuka.

TIP: This dish can be premade in the morning and eaten cold later in the day.

BEETS FRICASSEE

Ingredients

2 beets
½ yellow onion
2 tablespoons avocado oil
1 tablespoon herbs, any mixture of fennel seeds, dried rosemary, tarragon, oregano, basil, and savory
2 tablespoons parsley, chopped

Instructions

Peel the beets, rinse them, and slice them thinly. Also, peel and thinly slice the onion.

In a large skillet, heat the avocado oil to a medium temperature. Add the beets and onion, as well as the mixed herbs, to the pan. Sauté for 15–20 minutes.

Taste to check that the beets are fully cooked. If they are still crunchy, leave them to slow cook over low heat for a few more minutes.

Remove from heat. Plate. Add chopped parsley and serve immediately.

MUSHROOM SOUP

Ingredients

½ tablespoon extra-virgin olive oil
½ medium onion, white or yellow, diced
½ teaspoon garlic, minced
1 teaspoon dried oregano
1 teaspoon dried basil
2½ cups white button mushrooms, sliced
1¾ cups cremini mushrooms, sliced
1 large portobello mushroom, sliced
1 tablespoon tamari (or coconut liquid aminos)
7 ounces unsweetened coconut milk (canned)
High-quality salt, to taste
Black pepper, to taste
1–2 tablespoons fresh basil, chopped (optional), for garnish

Instructions

Add the olive oil to a soup pot along with the diced onion, minced garlic, and dried oregano and basil, and sauté over low heat, stirring occasionally, until the onion has softened and is translucent. This takes 2–3 minutes.

Add the sliced mushrooms and the tamari (or coconut aminos) to the pot, and cover it. Cook on medium high for around 10 minutes. This will allow the mushrooms to release their water. Stir occasionally.

After 10 minutes, remove the lid and cook for a further 10 minutes uncovered to allow some of the water to cook off.

Stir in the coconut milk and cook for a final 10 minutes, stirring occasionally, allowing the flavors to blend properly.

Season with salt and black pepper to taste.

Garnish with fresh basil and serve.

APPLE, ALMOND, AND ARUGULA SALAD WITH VINAIGRETTE

Vinaigrette Ingredients

⅓ cup extra-virgin olive oil
2 tablespoons white balsamic vinegar
1 tablespoon honey
2 teaspoons Dijon mustard
Salt and pepper, to taste

Salad Ingredients

1 medium green apple, cored and diced
2 tablespoons raw shallots, diced
2 tablespoons raw almonds, chopped
3 cups arugula, roughly chopped

Instructions for the Vinaigrette

Put the olive oil, vinegar, honey, and mustard in a jar with a lid. Shake until it is mixed well. Season with salt and pepper.

Instructions for Preparing the Salad

Cut the apple in half and scoop out the core. Dice the apple and shallots. Chop the almonds. Toss in a salad bowl with the arugula.

Divide the salad into two equal servings. Top each with 2 tablespoons of vinaigrette.

Fasting-Mimicking Dinners

GINGER CARROT SOUP

Ingredients

4 teaspoons extra-virgin olive oil
¼ cup chopped onion
1 tablespoon grated ginger
2 cloves garlic, minced
1 teaspoons ground coriander
¼ cup chopped almonds, about 24
3 cups carrots
16 ounces water (or vegetable stock)
1½ cups or ¾ can unsweetened, canned coconut milk
Salt, to taste (depending on salt content of stock)

Instructions

In a large soup pot, sauté the onions, ginger, garlic, coriander, and chopped almonds in olive oil over low heat until the onions soften and fragrance is emitted, about 2–3 minutes. Stir occasionally to avoid burning.

Chop the carrots into ¼-inch rounds. Add the carrots and water (or broth) to the soup pot, blending with a wooden spoon, and seasoning with salt, to taste.

Cook for about 20 minutes over medium heat, stirring occasionally, and then puree in a blender, in batches if necessary, until it reaches a desirable consistency.

Return to the pot and swirl in the coconut milk. Heat until warm.

Serve immediately.

PAD THAI

Sauce Ingredients

1 tablespoons almond butter
3 tablespoons unsweetened rice wine vinegar
3 tablespoon coconut liquid aminos
3 tablespoons honey
1½ tablespoons lime juice
1 tablespoon hot sauce or more, to taste (beware of sugar and other additives in hot sauce)
¼ teaspoon salt, or more, to taste

Stir-fry Ingredients

1 tablespoon extra-virgin olive oil
1 clove garlic, minced
2 cups zucchini, spiralized noodles (or cut into long, thin strips)
1 cup carrot, spiralized noodles (or cut into long, thin strips)
2 cups purple cabbage, sliced thinly

1 red Bell pepper, sliced into long, thin strips
3 scallions, chopped into 1-inch pieces
½ cup roasted sunflower seeds
1 tablespoons chopped cilantro
Lime wedges

Instructions for the Sauce

Add all the sauce ingredients (almond butter, rice wine vinegar, coconut aminos, honey, lime juice, hot sauce, and salt) to a medium-sized mixing bowl, whisking until well combined. Set aside.

Instructions for the Stir-fry

Heat a large skillet over high heat. Add the oil and garlic. Sauté for 5–7 minutes until softened and fragrant.

Add zucchini, carrots, red Bell pepper, scallions, and purple cabbage, stir-frying them for 4–5 minutes, until heated through and softening. Be careful, however, not to allow the noodles to get mushy. Overcooking vegetable noodles will result in a watery dish.

Remove pan from heat, pour the vegetable mixture into a bowl. Drizzle them with sauce, then toss to coat the vegetables.

Serve in bowls and garnish with sunflower seeds, cilantro, and lime wedges.

POTATOES AND VEGGIES WITH KALE PESTO

Pesto Ingredients

1 clove garlic
1 tablespoon pine nuts
5 ounces or 8 cups of loosely packed kale, stems removed
2 cups fresh basil leaves
2 tablespoon extra-virgin olive oil
Salt and pepper, to taste

Potatoes and Veggies Ingredients

9 ounces or 1⅛ cups potatoes, chopped into bite-sized chunks
2 teaspoons olive oil, divided
Salt and pepper, to taste
Pinch of red pepper flakes (optional)
10 ounces zucchini, sliced into¼-inch thick rounds

Instructions for the Pesto

Place garlic, pine nuts, kale, and basil in a food processor. Process until the mixture becomes like a paste. Slowly add olive oil and process until smooth. Add salt and pepper to taste. Set aside.

Instructions for the Potatoes and Veggies

Preheat the oven to 425°F/220°C. Toss the potatoes with 1 teaspoon olive oil. Season with salt, pepper, and red pepper flakes (if using). Roast the potatoes on a rimmed baking sheet for 30 minutes, or until tender.

Five minutes before the potatoes are done roasting, sauté zucchini rounds in the remaining 1 teaspoon olive oil for just a few minutes, until al dente. Remove from heat.

Toss potatoes, zucchini, and pesto together in a large bowl. Serve immediately.

VEGGIE HASH WITH LEEKS, CAULIFLOWER, AND ASPARAGUS

Ingredients

1 tablespoon extra-virgin olive oil
1 leek
½ onion
1 tablespoon grated fresh ginger
1 teaspoon chopped garlic
1 small head cauliflower, riced or chopped
1 large bunch asparagus, ends trimmed and roughly chopped
1 tablespoon chopped fresh herbs, like parsley, basil, and thyme
Salt and black pepper, to taste
4 tablespoons hemp seeds
Drizzle of olive oil or hemp oil (optional)

Instructions

Heat olive oil in a pan and sauté leek, onion, and ginger together, until fragrant and the onion is translucent.

Add the garlic and cauliflower and stir-fry for a couple of minutes.

Add the asparagus and cook for a few more minutes.

Add the fresh herbs, salt, and pepper.

Serve with a sprinkle of hemp seeds and a drizzle of olive oil or hemp seed oil.

CREAM OF BROCCOLI SOUP

Ingredients

½ cup onion, minced
1 garlic clove, minced
1 tablespoon extra-virgin olive oil
1½ cups potatoes, peeled and diced
1¾ cups broccoli florets, chopped
4 cups water
¼ cup almonds, coarsely chopped
¼ cup unsweetened coconut milk (from a carton)
Pepper, to taste
Fresh parsley sprigs, for garnish

Instructions

Finely chop the onion and garlic. Sauté with the olive oil for 2 minutes in the bottom of a soup pot.

Add the potatoes to the pot and sauté with the onion for another 5 minutes.

Divide broccoli florets into small pieces and add to the soup pot along with the water. Simmer for 20 minutes until the vegetables are cooked through.

Puree in a blender to the desired consistency.

Add the coconut milk and bring to a soft simmer, briefly.

Fold in the almonds and season with pepper, to taste.

Serve immediately and garnish with parsley.

CHAPTER TWELVE

Basic Recipes for a Healthy Lifestyle

Recipes that fall into this category include those for salad dressings, smoothies, fermented foods like sauerkraut and raw apple cider vinegar, antioxidant citrus "shots," yogurt, and sourdough bread. In other words, these are anti-inflammatory foods and beverages that you and your family will eat every day which may help keep the gut microbiome balanced, promote healthy skin, and taste delicious. Some of these have been referenced throughout the book.

Salad Dressing

SIMPLE, EVERYDAY "WING-IT" DRESSING

Ingredients

⅛ cup extra-virgin olive oil

⅛ cup apple cider vinegar (see p. 200)
1 heaping teaspoon honey
1 teaspoon Dijon mustard

Instructions

Whisk all the ingredients together and serve over salad or a power bowl.

TIP: You can substitute lemon juice or balsamic vinegar for the apple cider vinegar.

GREEN GODDESS DRESSING

Ingredients

1 cup whole milk yogurt from grass-fed cows
1 cup fresh parsley
1 cup mixed, soft, leafy herbs, like dill, mint, tarragon, and/or cilantro
2 tablespoons chopped chives
2 tablespoons fresh lemon juice, plus ½ teaspoon zest
1 tablespoon extra-virgin olive oil
2 teaspoons capers (high in antioxidants)
1 garlic clove
¼ teaspoon sea salt
Freshly ground black pepper

Instructions

Combine all the ingredients and blend in food processor. Serve with salad, in a power bowl, or as a condiment.

Fermented Foods

SAUERKRAUT

I love sauerkraut as a lifestyle recipe because it can be used multiple times per week as a condiment or plate accompaniment. Purchasing it is fine, but if you're inclined to make your own, it's very much worth the work since it will keep for several weeks in the fridge and you know exactly what's in it.

The fresher the cabbage, the more juice it will produce. This will enable you to make a sufficient amount of brine to reach the top of the container. The finished sauerkraut will also have a much better texture. Avoid using iodized salt because it will interfere with the fermentation process.

NOTE: I recommend using a ceramic crock pot for fermentation or half-gallon or gallon glass jars. Some people like to ferment their kraut in plastic buckets, but these days the concern for microplastic exposure should deter us from fermenting anything in plastic.

Ingredients

1½–2 teaspoons sea salt for every pound of cabbage (but not iodized salt)*

1 pound very fresh green cabbage, shredded into small pieces with a grater or very finely shredded with a knife.

Instructions

PACKING THE CABBAGE: Mix the cabbage with the salt (as directed above). Transfer the pieces of shredded cabbage to a glass jar or ceramic crockpot a bit at a time and mash them down with a tamper. (I use a large wooden ladle.) Fill the jar only to about two-thirds full, as the cabbage will bubble as it ferments and could overflow if you do not leave sufficient room.

Continue to tamp down the cabbage, releasing more juice, until the cabbage is completely submerged under brine naturally produced by pressing on the cabbage and any air pockets in the cabbage pieces have been removed. (This is important for preventing mold growth.)

If you've mashed all you can mash and you still do"t have enough brine to cover the cabbage you'll need to make some supplemental liquid that is consistent with the salinity of the cabbage brine: Dissolve 1 teaspoon salt in 1 cup water (creating a 2-percent solution of salt water) and add this to the jar until the cabbage is completely submerged under the liquid.

The cabbage must remain submerged under the brine during fermentation, which takes a few weeks. I like to place the outer leaves of the cabbage (the leaves you remove to get to the tender portion) on top of the shredded and submerged cabbage in order to prevent air pockets. Place clean rocks or weights on top of the outer leaves to keep the contents submerged.

FERMENTING YOUR SAUERKRAUT: Place the jar of cabbage and brine in a dark place that is between 65–70F (18–21C), the ideal temperature for fermenting.

Most recipes call for allowing the kraut to ferment for two to three weeks, but an old man of my acquaintance who's been making the most amazing sauerkraut for the past four decades specifically instructed me to let mine sit for six weeks. The outcome has been a perfectly fermented and delicious sauerkraut.

After four days of fermenting, start tasting the cabbage daily until it reaches your desired texture and level of tanginess. Don't be alarmed if the brine becomes fizzy, this is completely normal and a positive sign of microbial activity.

NOTE: If you're not using an airlock lid be sure to open the lid of your jar/crock every day to release the pressure and "burp" your kraut. This will prevent an over-pressurized jar from bursting.

The color of the cabbage will change from green to a pale yellowish beige.

STORING YOUR SAUERKRAUT: Once your sauerkraut has reached the level of tanginess that you desire, it's time to screw the lid on tight (remove the airlock lid if using and replace it with a regular lid). If using a crock, it's time to move the kraut to mason jars and process appropriately.

Store the sauerkraut in the fridge or a cold cellar (storage temperature should be between 38–50F/3–10C).

Fermentation won't stop but it will be greatly slowed down.

If you haven't processed your kraut in a water bath for preservation, stored in the fridge the sauerkraut will keep for many months. If your sauerkraut is too salty for your taste simply give it a rinse before eating.

Eat your sauerkraut raw to reap the benefits of the probiotics or use it in any recipe calling for sauerkraut.

HOMEMADE APPLE CIDER VINEGAR

The best time to make a batch of apple cider vinegar is right after you have made applesauce or baked an apple pie. Reserve the cores and peels. This recipe uses only three ingredients.

NOTE: On different occasions, I have used a one-quart mason jar, a half-gallon jar, and a full gallon jar depending on the quantity of my apple discards. Adjust your measures to match.

Ingredients

Apple peels and cores, enough to fill just over half of your fermenting vessel

Sugar: 1 tablespoon per 1 cup of water (or 1 cup per 1 gallon water)

Filtered water

Instructions

Gather collected apple scraps and add them to your jar (or other fermenting vessel) until it is filled just over halfway.

Pour lukewarm filtered water over the apples into the container until it is almost full, reserving space for the sugar; as you do, measure the total amount of water you've added.

Stir in sugar (in the ratio listed above).

Optional: Add a splash of a finished organic apple cider vinegar (even a store-bought brand) to inoculate the culture in your jar and encourage fermenting.

Stir the combined ingredients until thoroughly mixed, and cover the vessel with cheesecloth or breathable fabric. It needs exposure to air. *Note:* Fruit flies love this concoction so you may want to seal the edge of the fabric with a rubberband.

Store the jug in a dark location at a temperature of around 70–75°F/21–23°C for two weeks to ferment, stirring it regularly to prevent mold from forming on top. If needed, add another layer of material, like a dark towel, on top of the container to block out light.

After two weeks, strain the liquid from the fermenting vessel into a similar sized storage container and cover again to reserve it. Compost the spent fruit.

Move the covered container of liquid to a location that is out of the way, where long-term it may continue fermentation, and maintain the darkness. A cooler room temperature at this stage is okay, but do not refrigerate the vinegar yet.

After one month, sample the vinegar to see if it is finished fermenting and tart enough for your liking. If needed, allow it to continue to ferment for a total of two to three months.

Once it has fermented to your desired flavor and tartness, transfer the apple cider vinegar into bottles with lids (or swing top bottles). Store in the refrigerator, and enjoy!

WHOLE-GRAIN SOURDOUGH BREAD

As discussed in Chapter 6, "Inflammatory Foods," not all grains or breads are created the same. Mass-produced breads are problematic and may exacerbate our health issues because they're made very quickly (with no time for fermentation), they use grains grown with glyphosate, which are then highly processed into flour, and then they're finished with harmful oils, sugars, and preservatives added to extend their shelf life. Bread as a superfood dates back to 10,000 years ago, but this kind of bread isn't it.

My favorite whole-grain sourdough bread recipe is one that my family eats almost every morning *and* it's so good it's practically life changing. To paraphrase something I recently read: Everything else tastes like cake!

The most unusual ingredient is the "starter." Ask around in your community, especially if you know foodies who like to bake. Most bakers would be glad to give you a bit that you can feed and nurture in your home. Also see the Resources section for a mail-order option. I've also included trustworthy sources for flour made from specialty grains.

Ingredients

2 cups filtered water
2 cups of active sourdough starter (see Resources)
4 teaspoons high-quality salt, such as Himalayan salt, sea salt, or Redmond Real® Salt
6 cups of organic whole-grain flour, made from spelt, red winter wheat, Sonora wheat, or einkorn (see Resources)

Instructions

Combine the sourdough starter, water, and salt in a large bowl. Stir and let stand for 5 minutes.

Start adding flour gradually. Begin with 2 cups of the whole-grain flour and let it sit for 5 minutes. The reason for this is that whole-grain flour absorbs water slowly. You want to give the flour time to absorb the moisture otherwise you will be tempted to add too much flour and the dough ball will become very dense and unpleasant.

Add the remaining 4 cups of flour one cup at a time with a 5-minute rest in between. I like to use a large plastic spoon for mixing dough because the plastic doesn't stick quite as much as wood, unlike wood, and is easier to clean. The consistency you're looking for ultimately is a ball of dough that holds its shape without flattening right away.

Over the course of the next ninety minutes, please stretch and fold your bread two to three times. Instructions for the stretch and fold can be found at Breadtopia.com.

Once all the flour has been added, let your dough sit in the cleaned bowl at room temperature to rise. Depending on the temperature of your home, this rising phase will take 8–12 hours. Leaving the dough to rise overnight works well. If your dough has expanded and looks puffy with an inflated dome, you know you have a perfect rise. If the dome looks fermented and bubbly but flattened, it most likely overrose and will still make a wonderful bread but not quite as fluffy. This is something that requires experimentation because it's slightly different every time.

After this first overnight rise, heavily flour a countertop and pour the dough onto the floured surface. At this point, your dough will be so sticky that you won't be able to shape it with your hands. A bench scraper will be a great tool for working with the dough effectively, but a pastry knife works well also. The goal now is to shape the dough back into a ball as best you can, and set it back into a new bowl or the same bowl which has been cleaned. (I use a Banneton proofing basket, which is designed specifically for sourdough). The shape of the bowl will determine the shape of your loaf.

Place the bowl or basket in a plastic bag and allow for the second rise to take 3–5 hours. Use the classic finger dent test to check for "doneness." Push your fingertip into the dough and if it bounces back right away, but not all the way, it is considered perfect. If it bounces back all the way, the dough is over proofed; and if the dough doesn't bounce back at all, it is under-proofed and just needs more time.

Before baking the bread, preheat your oven to 550°F/288°C. I like to use a clay baker (see Resources). If you don't have a clay baker, you can use a Dutch oven. Preheat the clay baker or Dutch oven in your hot oven for 40 minutes before you put the wet dough into it.

When the oven and baker are ready, take your dough and invert it onto your floured counter again. Pull the baker out of the oven and place a small amount of cornmeal or flour at the bottom of the baker to prevent the dough from sticking.

Place the dough in the baker and cover with the preheated lid right away. Place the lidded baker in the oven and immediately take the temperature down to 450°F/232°C. Bake for 40 minutes.

Remove the lid and bake for an additional 15 minutes at 350°F/176°C.

Let bread cool completely before cutting (the most difficult part of the process).

ENJOY!

HOMEMADE YOGURT

At first blush, making yogurt may seem tedious, but I assure you that it most definitely isn't. It's so simple, in fact, that it takes less than two minutes of hands-on time to prepare a batch once you have the routine down.

I began making yogurt at home years ago, using Ben Greenfield's recipe from his book *Boundless Cooking*. Ben is specific about the particular probiotic strains he uses to ferment his yogurt, two kinds of *Lactobacillus reuteri,* which he selected because of robust data about their benefits to the skin (promoting collagen production and elasticity), hormone balance, bone health, and overall antiaging and healing. I no longer make it exactly the way he does; I've adapted it to the equipment in my kitchen and the proportions I like to eat and use throughout the week. You should adapt this recipe for your own needs, too.

Eating homemade yogurt at least a few times per week is good for maintaining our gut health. It can be substituted for sour cream, mayo (sometimes), and buttermilk in a salad dressing. Try serving it with berries or an apple.

First, you need to make a yogurt starter. This requires a twenty-four-hour-long process of fermentation. After that, you can make new batches of yogurt by adding a few tablespoons of starter to fresh cream or milk. Below are instructions for both the starter and subsequent batches.

Ingredients for Yogurt Starter

1 quart grass-fed cream, whole cow's milk, goat milk, sheep milk, or canned full-fat coconut milk, divided
1 tablespoon organic inulin powder (a prebiotic)

10 tablets unflavored Gastrus by BioGaia, crushed (or capsules that have been emptied of their contents)

Instructions for Yogurt Starter

In a large glass jar (I use a mason jar with a plastic lid), combine 2 tablespoons of your milk or cream of choice with the inulin and the prebiotic and thoroughly mix them. Add the remaining milk of choice or cream and give the jar a good shake.

At this juncture, you need to allow the starter to ferment in a warm place for twenty-four hours undisturbed. There are several ways to keep it warm without overheating it and killing the beneficial bacteria. You need them alive to convert the lactase in the cream.

Way 1. I place mine in a food dehydrator at 110° F/43° C.

Way 2. Put your starter in a yogurt maker.

Way 3. Put the jar on a heating pad (set on low).

Way 4. Put the jar in an oven with the light on, or on the "proofing" setting (as long as the temperature reads between 110 and 115° F/43 and 46°C.

After the mixture ferments for approximately twenty-four hours, shake the jar gently and place it in the refrigerator. That is your starter, which is thinner than the yogurt most of us like to eat. This is normal. Feel free to consume it like you would any other yogurt.

Instructions for Subsequent Batches

Make your next batch of yogurt using 2–3 tablespoons of the starter yogurt, 1 quart of milk or cream, 1 tablespoon of inulin, and only 1 tablet (or capsule) of Gastrus.

Ferment as you did before. As long as you keep feeding the *L. reuteri* bacteria with milk and inulin, and do not overheat it, it will stay alive and multiply indefinitely. I personally, add a capsule of the probiotic strain to every batch I make.

Smoothies and Shots

BERRY KEFIR SMOOTHIE

Ingredients

1½ cups frozen mixed berries
1 cup plain kefir
½ medium banana
2 teaspoons almond butter
½ teaspoon vanilla extract
1 tablespoon cacao nibs (optional)

Instructions

Combine all ingredients in a blender, with the exception of the cacao nibs, and blend until smooth. Once these ingredients are smoothly blended, add cacao nibs and pulse the blender briefly to retain some of their crunchy texture.

TIP: If using *fresh* berries, add a cup of ice to ensure cold satisfaction.

GREEN SMOOTHIE

Ingredients

4–6 cups dark leafy greens (parsley, spinach, or kale)
1–1½ cups water or coconut water
4 stalks of Swiss chard
1 whole apple
1 banana
2 tablespoon hemp seeds
1 cup berries (blackberries, blueberries, or raspberries)
1 cup ice

Instructions

Blend all ingredients in a blender. Enjoy.

TURMERIC GINGER LEMON SHOTS

Ingredients

1 small orange (for sweetness)
2 small lemons
¼ cup chopped fresh turmeric (peeling optional)
¼ cup chopped fresh ginger (peeling optional)
⅛ teaspoon fresh black pepper (helps your body assimilate the turmeric)
¼ teaspoon extra-virgin olive oil or coconut oil (optional: to help improve turmeric absorption)

Instructions

Juice the ingredients in a juicer and then shake the resulting juice vigorously in a shaker with ice. Pour out 2–3individual shots and serve them immediately.

If you don't have a juicer, you can use a high-speed blender but the juice will have more of a gritty texture.

TIP: If you like tartness, add another lemon and omit the orange.

AFTERWORD

As you plunge into your healing journey, you likely feel excited, nervous, and in the need of some courage for the three months ahead. Take a breath and trust in the process. In a world of immediate access and the promise of quick, effortless results, your dedication to yourself is commendable and your vision for healing is already creating change.

Easily and naturally remind yourself that your body is a self-healing organism just waiting to grace you with the beauty you were born with.

With immense gratitude,
Dr. Anik

ACKNOWLEDGMENTS

I spent two decades avoiding my previous life with psoriasis. I believed that if I looked back, I would create the vulnerability for it to return. However I now realize that the only way forward is to understand and empower as many people as I can who are suffering like I did.

A few years ago, I shared my story with a group while attending a seminar. Hearing and seeing the responses from the attendees—who told me they were not only inspired by my story themselves but also all knew at least one other person with psoriasis who was suffering to no avail—helped me to realize that I could no longer keep this part of my life to myself. For these reasons, I would first like to express gratitude for the strangers in that conference room.

I've spent over two decades working in a profession which trusts that the body has an innate ability to heal and that, with time and consistency of effort, extraordinary healing can occur. My first chiropractor, the late Dr. Thomas Lindsay, lovingly set me on this path and I am forever grateful for his guidance. Each week, I have the privilege of meeting with chiropractic friends who have held me accountable and who repeatedly reminded me that I was meant to write this book. For this, thank you Dr. Jenny Bruck, Dr. Stephanie Mills Ryan, and Dr. Jeremy Meadows.

I was honored to work with my brilliant editor, Stephanie Gunning, who was patiently hypervigilant and always found the right questions to ask, never missing a contradiction or an extra comma.

Finally, I thank my loving family, including my newly found sister, Cathy, and my parents, Gilles and Lise, who have always been deeply entrenched in my journey. A big thank you to my sons, Simon and Marco, who have made my motherhood dreams come true. I've dedicated this book to my amazing husband, who for twenty-five years has always reminded me of my beauty.

END NOTES

Introduction

1. Kris Martins. “What Is an Autoimmune Disease?” WebMD.com (October 21, 2025).
2. Colleen De Bellefonds. “Newborns and Rice Cereal: Is It Safe to Give Rice Cereal to a Baby Under Four Months?” TheBump.com (October 23, 2025).

PART ONE: BACKGROUND

Chapter 1: Medical Definitions

1. National Psoriasis Foundation. “About Psoriatic Arthritis,” Psorisis.org (accessed January 21, 2026).
2. Ibid.
3. “What Is a Keratinocyte Cell and What Is Its Function?” BiologyInsights.com (July 25, 2025).
4. National Psoriasis Foundation.
5. Ibid.

Chapter 2: Your Genes Are Not Your Destiny

1. Hani A. AlShobaili, Muhammad Shahzad, Abdullah Al-Marshood, et al. “Genetic Background of Psoriasis,” *International Journal of Health Sciences,* vol. 4, no. 1 (January 2010): pp. 23–9.
2. National Human Genome Research Institute. “The Human Genome Project,” Genome.gov (accessed

January 30, 2026). There is an excellent glossary on this website that offers extensive definitions of terms like *gene* and *base pair*.

3. Press release. "Number of Genes in Human Genome Lower than Previously Estimated," News.MIT.edu (October 29, 2004).
4. National Human Genome Research Institute. "2000: Drosophila and Arabidopsis Genomes Sequenced," Genome.gov (accessed January 21, 2026).
5. John Cloud. "Why Your DNA Isn't Your Destiny," *Time* (January 6, 2010).
6. Shelley L. Berger, Tony Kouzarides, Ramin Sheikhattar, et al. "An Operational Definition of Epigenetics," *Genes Development*, vol. 23, no. 7 (April 1, 2009): pp. 781–3.

Chapter 3: Commonly Prescribed Drugs

1. Jessica T. DeFrank, Nancy D. Berkman, Leila Kahwati, et al. "Direct-to-Consumer Advertising of Prescription Drugs and the Patient–Prescriber Encounter: A Systematic Review," *Health Communication*, vol. 35, no. 6 (May 2020): pp. 739–46.
2. April W. Armstrong, Menan D. Mehta, Calyton W. Schupp, et al. "Psoriasis Prevalence in Adults in the United States," *JAMA Dermatology*, vol. 157, no. 8 (June 30, 2021): pp. 940–6.
3. Andrea Park. "AbbVie's Skyrizi Takes Full-Year TV Ad Spending Crown Yet Again, with J&J's Tremfya in Hot Pursuit," FiercePharma.com (January 16, 2026).
4. Abstract of a report released on May 4, 2026: *Psoriasis Treatment Market Size, Share & Industry Analysis, By Drug*

Class (TNF Inhibitors, Interleukins Inhibitors, and Others), By Type (Plaque Psoriasis, Psoriatic Arthritis, and Others), By Product Type (Biologics and Non-Biologics), By Route of Administration (Oral, Parenteral/Systemic, and Topical), By Distribution Channel (Hospital Pharmacies, Retail Pharmacies, and Online Pharmacies), and Regional Forecast, 2026-2034, FortunebusinessInsights.com (accessed May 19, 2026).

5. Psoriasis and Psoriatic Arthritis Alliance. "Steroids," PAPAA.org (accessed January 21, 2026).
6. American Academy of Dermatology Association. "Psoriasis Treatment: Corticosteroids You Apply to the Skin," AAD.org (accessed January 21, 2026).
7. Lisa H. Lam and Jeffrey L. Sugarman. "Adrenal Suppression with Chronic Topical Corticosteroid Use in Psoriasis Patients," *Journal of Drugs in Dermatology,* vol. 15, no. 8 (August 1, 2016): pp. 945–8.
8. Johns Hopkins Medicine. "Adrenal Glands," HopkinsMedicine.org (accessed January 21, 2026).
9. Anna A Kasperlik-Załuska, Barbara Zarnocka, and Wlodzimierz Czech. "Autoimmunity as the Most Frequent Cause of Idiopathic Secondary Adrenal Insufficiency: Report of 111 Cases," *Journal of Autoimmunity,* vol. 36, no. 3 (May 2003): pp. 155–9.
10. Grace K. Kim. "The Rationale Behind Topical Vitamin D Analogs in the Treatment of Psoriasis," *Journal of Clinical and Aesthetic Dermatology,* vol. 3, no.8 (August 2010): pp. 46–53.
11. National Psoriasis Foundation. "Methotrexate," Psoriasis.org (accessed January 21, 2026).

12. Rashmi Dhital and Arthur Kavanaugh. "Autoimmune Consequences of Biologics," *Journal of Allergy and Clinical Immunology,* vol. 149, no. 1 (January 2022): pp. 48–50.
13. Ibid.
14. National Psoriasis Foundation. "Biologics," Psioriasis.org (accessed January 21, 2026). Also see, AbbVie Biotechnology Ltd. "Humira: Adalimumab," humira.com (accessed January 21, 2026); and Janssen Biotech, Inc. "Remicade: Infliximab," remicade.com (accessed January 21, 2026).
15. Jason J. Emer, Amylynne Frankel, and Joshua A. Zeichner. "A Practical Approach to Monitoring Patients on Biological Agents for the Treatment of Psoriasis," *Journal of Clinical and Aesthetic Dermatology,* vol. 3, no. 8 (August 2010): pp. 20–6.
16. Victoria Ruffing. "Side Effects of Biologic Medications," Johns Hopkins Arthritis Center (January 12, 2016).
17. National Toxicology Program. "Coal Tars and Coal-Tar Pitches: CAS No. 8007-45-2 (Coal Tar)," *Fifteenth Report on Carcinogens* (December 21, 2021) [Internet].

Chapter 4: Four Key Causes of Autoimmunity

1. Sharon Baughman Shively, Braxton B. Wannamaker, Adam M. Willis, et al. "Editorial: Traumatic Brain Injury and Autoimmune Disease," *Frontiers in Neurology* (June 17, 2021).
2. Magda Havas. "Precursors Need to Be Considered to Promote Recovery from Idiopathic Environmental Intolerance—Attributed to Electromagnetic Fields,"

Medical Research Archives (European Society of Medicine), vol. 13, no. 1 (January 31, 2025): online.

3. D. Bonciani, C. Della Bella, A. Corrà, et al. "The Impact of Antibiotic Therapy in Psoriasis Patients with Active Streptococcal Infection: A Prospective Study," *Journal of Dermatology,* vol. 52, no. 3 (February 3, 2025): pp. 432–8.
4. Winston E. Anthony, Bin Wang, Kimberley Sukhum, et. al. "Acute and Persistent Effects of Commonly Used Antibiotics on the Gut Microbiome and Resistome in Healthy Adults," *Cell Reports,* vol. 39, no. 2 (April 12, 2022): p. 110649.
5. Shahrose Rahman, Amber L. O'Connor, Sarah L. Becker, et. al. "Gut Microbial Metabolites and Its Impact on Human Health," *Annals of Gastroenterology,* vol. 36, no. 4 (May 29, 2023): pp. 360–8.
6. Grace K Kim and James Q. Del Rosso. "Drug-Provoked Psoriasis: Is It Drug Induced or Drug Aggravated? Understanding Pathophysiology and Clinical Relevance," *Journal of Clinical and Aesthetic Dermatology,* vol. 3, no. 1 (January 2010): pp. 32–8.
7. Fang-Yih Liaw, Wei-Liang Chen, Tung-Wei Kao, et al "Exploring the Link Between Cadmium and Psoriasis in a Nationally Representative Sample," *Scientific Reports,* vol. 7, no. 1 (May 11, 2-17): 1723.
8. Ibid.
9. Di Zhao, Atul Aravindakshan, Markus Hilpert, et al. "Metal/Metalloid Levels in Electronic Cigarette Liquids, Aerosols, and Human Biosamples: A Systematic Review,"

Environmental Health Perspectives, vol. 128, no. 3 (March 2020): 36001.

10. Grace K Kim and James Q. Del Rosso. "Drug-Provoked Psoriasis: Is It Drug Induced or Drug Aggravated?" *Journal of Clinical Aesthetic Dermatology*, vol. 3, no. 1 (January 2010): pp. 32–8.
11. Samina Shaikh [Letter to the Editor]. "NSAIDs: Unveiling Their Role in Drug-Induced Psoriasis," *Psoriasis: Targets and Therapy* (September 13, 2024): pp. 101–2.
12. Vanessa M. Awad, Sirisha Sakhamuru, Srikala Kambampati, et al. "Mechanisms of Beta-Blocker Induced Psoriasis, and Psoriasis De Novo at the Cellular Level," *Cureus*, vol. 12, no. 7 (July 2, 2020): e8964.
13. Deepak M. Balak and Enes Hajdarbegovic. "Drug-induced Psoriasis: Clinical Perspectives," *Journal of Psoriasis and Psoriatic Arthritis*, vol. 7 (December 7, 2017): pp. 87–94.
14. Gonjin Song, Ji Yea Kim, Ha Young Yoon, et al. "A Systematic Review and Meta-Analysis of Angiotensin-Converting Enzyme Inhibitor Use and Psoriasis Incidence," *Scientific Reports*, vol. 11 (May 11, 2021): 10037.
15. Hanjiang Gu, Yufei Zhang, Weihui Zeng, et al. "Participation of Interferons in Psoriatic Inflammation," *Cytokine & Growth Factor Reviews*, vol. 64, (April 2022): pp. 12–20. Also *see*, M. Afshar, A.D. Martinez, R.L. Gallo, et al. "Induction and Exacerbation of Psoriasis with Interferon-Alpha Therapy for Hepatitis C: A Review and Analysis of 36 Cases," *Journal of the European Academy of Dermatology and Venereology*, vol. 27 (June 1, 2012): pp. 771–8.

16. "H.R. 5546: National Childhood Vaccine Injury Act of 1986," Congress.gov (accessed January 21, 2026). Passed by the 99th Congress (1985–1986).
17. Health Resources and Services Administration. "National Vaccine Injury Compensation Program," HRSA.gov (accessed February 24, 2026).
18. P.W. Newacheck, P.P. Budetti, and N. Halfon. "Trends in Activity-Limiting Chronic Conditions among Children." *American Journal of Public Health,* vol. 76, no. 2 (February 1986): pp. 178–84. Also see, "Managing Chronic Health Conditions," CDC.gov (July 9, 2024).
19. Adam Rowden. "What to Know about Vaccines and Psoriasis," *Medical News Today* (September 29, 2021). For insights specific to Covid-19 vaccines, also *see,* Luca Potestio, Teresa Battista, Sara Cacciapuoti, et. al. "New Onset and Exacerbation of Psoriasis Following COVID-19 Vaccination: A Review of the Current Knowledge," *Biomedicines,* vol. 11, no. 8 (August 3, 2023): 2191.
20. Azhar Choudhry, Julie Mathena, Jessica D. Albano, et. al. "Safety Evaluation of Adenovirus Type 4 and Type 7 Attenuated Vaccine Live, Oral in Military Recruits," *Vaccine,* vol. 34, no. 38 (August 31, 2016). pp. 3558–64.
21. GlaxoSmithKline Biologicals. "Package Insert for Infanrix," FDA.gov (accessed January 21, 2026).
22. Sanofi Pasteur Inc. "Package insert for Daptacel," FDA.gov (accessed January 21, 2026).
23. Teva Pharmaceuticals USA, Inc. "Package insert for Adenovirus Type 4 and Type 7 Vaccine, Live, Oral," FDA.gov (accessed January 21, 2026).

24. Healthcare Providers. "Smallpox: Contraindications to Vaccination," CDC.gov (November 4, 2024).
25. Emmanouil Karampinis, Myrto-Maria Papadopoulou, Kleoniki Chaidaki, et. al. "Plaque Psoriasis Exacerbation and COVID-19 Vaccination: Assessing the Characteristics of the Flare and the Exposome Parameters," *Vaccines,* vol. 12, no. 2 (February 9, 2024): p.178.
26. Merck Sharp & Dohme LLC. "Package Insert for Measles, Mumps, and Rubella Virus Vaccine Live," FDA.gov (accessed January 21,2026).
27. Merck Sharp & Dohme LLC. "Package Insert for Gardasil," FDA.gov (accessed January 21, 2026).
28. Merck Sharp & Dohme LLC. "Package Insert for Measles, Mumps, and Rubella Virus Vaccine Live" FDA.gov (accessed January 21, 2026).
29. Ibid.
30. Sayaka Yoneyama, Koji Kamiya, Megumi Kishimoto, et al. "Generalized Exacerbation of Psoriasis Vulgaris Induced by Pneumococcal Polysaccharide Vaccine," *Journal of Dermatology,* vol. 46, no. 11 (November 2019): e442–3.
31. Jamie Eske. "What Is an MTHFR Gene Mutation?" MedicalNewsToday.com (August 21, 2025).
32. Muzeyyen Izmirli, Bilge Bulbul Sen, Eminenur Rifaioglu, et al. "Methylenetetrahydrofolate Reductase (MTHFR) C677T Polymorphism in Psoriasis in Southern Turkey," *Anais Brasilieros Dermatologia,* vol. 91, no. 5 (September–October 2016): pp. 611–3.

33. Matt Sommers. "MTHFR Mutation Gene Test: What You Need to Know," ClarityXDNA.com (May 19, 2025). Also *see,* Daniel Leclerc, Sahar Sibani, and Rima Rozen. "Molecular Biology of Methylenetetrahydrofolate Reductase (MTHFR) and Overview of Mutations/ Polymorphisms," Madame Curie Bioscience Database [Internet] (Austin, TX.: Landes Bioscience, 2000–2013); Ercan Karabacak, Ersin Aydin, Omer Ozcan, et al. "Methylenetetrahydrofolate Reductase (MTHFR) 677C>T Gene Polymorphism as a Possible Factor for Reducing Clinical Severity of Psoriasis," *International Journal of Clinical and Experimental Medicine,* vol. 7, no. 3 (2014): pp. 697–702; and Shanel Raghubeer and Tandi E. Matsha. "Methylenetetrahydrofolate (MTHFR), the One-Carbon Cycle, and Cardiovascular Risks," *Nutrients,* vol. 13, no. 12 (December 20, 2021): 4562.

34. Rachel B. Johnson. "Methylation 101: What Is It and Why Does It Matter for Health?" CASI.org (December 22, 2025).

35. Martin Beranek, Andrea Malkova, Zdenek Fiala, et al. "Goeckerman Therapy of Psoriasis: Genotoxicity, Dietary Micronutrients, Homocysteine, and MTHFR Gene Polymorphisms," *International Journal of Molecular Sciences,* vol. 20, no. 8 (April 17, 2019): 1908. Also *see,* Johann E. Gudjonsson and Gerald Krueger. "A Role for Epigenetics in Psoriasis: Methylated Cytosine–Guanine Sites Differentiate Lesional from Nonlesional Skin and from Normal Skin," *Journal of Investigative Dermatology,* vol.132, no. 3, pt. 1 (March 2012): pp. 506–8.

36. Martin Beranek, Andrea Malkova, Zdenek Fiala, et al. "Goeckerman Therapy of Psoriasis: Genotoxicity, Dietary Micronutrients, Homocysteine, and MTHFR Gene Polymorphisms," *International Journal of Molecular Sciences,* vol. 20, no. 8 (April 17, 2019): 1908. Also *see,* Johann E. Gudjonsson and Gerald Krueger. "A Role for Epigenetics in Psoriasis: Methylated Cytosine–Guanine Sites Differentiate Lesional from Nonlesional Skin and from Normal Skin," *Journal of Investigative Dermatology,* vol.132, no. 3, pt. 1 (March 2012): pp. 506–8.
37. Vaccine Safety. "Adjuvants and Vaccines," CDC.gov (December 20, 2024).
38. Tianli Tang and Yimeng Wang, Chao Wang, et. al. "Acetaminophen Exposure Alters the DNA Methylation Pattern of *Mugilogobius chulae,* along with the Changes in the Nrf2-Keap1 Signaling Pathway," *Comparative Biochemistry and Physiology,* vol. 270 (August 2023): 109655.
39. Laurie Rousset and Bruno Halioua. "Stress and Psoriasis," *International Journal of Dermatology,* vol. 57, no. 10 (October 2018): pp. 1165–72.
40. Doug Irving. *Chronic Conditions in America: Price and Prevalence.* rand.org (July 12, 2017).
41. J. Kiecolt-Glaser, T.J Loving, J.R. Stowell, et al. "Hostile Marital Interactions, Proinflammatory Cytokine Production, and Wound Healing," *Archives of General Psychiatry,* vol. 62, no. 12 (2005): pp.1377–84.
42. Erin Bartholomew. "Mindfulness and Meditation for Psoriasis: A Systematic Review," *Journal of Dermatologic Therapy,* vol. 12 (October 2022).

Chapter 5: Gut Health and the Microbiome

1. Lihui Chen, Jie Li, Wu Zhu, et al. "Skin and Gut Microbiome in Psoriasis: Gaining Insight Into the Pathophysiology of It and Finding Novel Therapeutic Strategies," *Frontiers in Microbiology,* vol. 11 (December 15, 2020): 589726. Also *see,* Jonathan R. Brestoff and David Artis. "Commensal Bacteria at the Interface of Host Metabolism and the Immune System," *Natural Immunology,* vol. 14, no. 7 (July 2013): pp. 676–84.
2. Mihaela C. Buhas, Laura I. Gavrilas, Rares Candrea, et. al. "Gut Microbiota in Psoriasis," *Nutrients,* vol. 14, no. 14 (July 20, 2022): 2970.
3. "Earth Microbiome Project," EarthMicrobiome.UCSD.edu (accessed January 22, 2026).
4. Video from *The Secret Word Inside You* Exhibition. "Building Your Microbiome from Birth," AMNH.org (accessed March 12, 2026).
5. Robert J Boyle, Despo Ierodiakonou, Tasnia Khan, et. al. "Hydrolysed Formula and Risk of Allergic or Autoimmune Disease: Systematic Review and Meta-Analysis," *BMJ,* vol. 352 (March 8, 2016): i974.
6. Ling Xiao, Belinda Van't Land, Phillip A. Engen, et al. "Human Milk Oligosaccharides Protect Against the Development of Autoimmune Diabetes in NOD-Mice," *Scientific Reports,* vol. 8, no. 1 (March 1, 2018): 3829.
7. Anastasia A. Theodosiou, Christine E. Jones, Robert C. Read, et al. "Microbiotoxicity: Antibiotic Usage and Its Unintended Harm to the Microbiome," *Current Opinion in*

Infectious Diseases, vol. 36, no. 5 (October 2023): pp. 371–8.

8. Ibid.
9. Ibid.
10. Patrik Lundquist, Eva Hagforsen, Michael Wagner, et. al. "Mild to Mild-to-Moderate Psoriasis Is Associated with Subclinical Inflammation in the Duodenum and a Tendency of Disturbed Intestinal Barrier," *Biochimica et Biophysica Acta,* vol. 1871, no. 3 (March 2025): 167634.
11. Bonggi Lee, Kyoung Mi Moon, and Choon Young Kim. "Tight Junction in the Intestinal Epithelium: Its Association with Diseases and Regulation by Phytochemicals," *Journal of Immunology Research,* vol. 11 (December 16, 2018): pp.1–11.

PART TWO: FOUNDATIONS OF A HEALTHY, WELL-STABILIZED LIFESTYLE

Chapter 6: Inflammatory Foods

1. This article was also published in print: Anahad O'Connor. "Sugar Backers Paid to Shift Blame to Fat," *New York Times* (September 13, 2016): section A, p. 1.
2. Aparna Shil, Luisa Maria Ladeira Faria, Caray Anne Walker, et al. "The Artificial Sweetener Neotame Negatively Regulates the Intestinal Epithelium Directly Through T1R3-Signaling and Indirectly Through Pathogenic Changes to Model Gut Bacteria," *Frontiers in Nutrition,* vol. 11 (April 23, 2024).
3. Liping Wang, Tiantian Ji, Ye Yuan, et al. "High-Fructose Corn Syrup Promotes Proinflammatory Macrophage

Activation via ROS-Mediated NF-κB Signaling and Exacerbates Colitis in Mice," *International Immunopharmacology,* vol. 109 (August 2022): 108814.

4. Ladan Afifi, Melissa J. Danesh, Kristina M. Lee, et al. "Dietary Behaviors in Psoriasis: Patient-Reported Outcomes from a U.S. National Survey," *Dermatology and Therapy,* vol. 7, no. 2 (June 2017): pp. 227–42.
5. Melissa Waddell. "The GMO High-Risk List: Canola," NonGMOProject.org (January 16, 2024).
6. Jean Mboma, Nadine Leblanc, Paul Angers, et al. "Effects of Cyclic Fatty Acid Monomers from Heated Vegetable Oil on Markers of Inflammation and Oxidative Stress in Male Wistar Rats," *Journal of Agricultural and Food Chemistry,* vol. 66, no. 27 (July 11, 2018): pp. 7172–80.
7. "Trusted Legal Help for People Harmed by Defective Drugs and Medical Devices," DrugWatch.com (accessed February 16, 2026).
8. Joanna K. Winstone, Khyatiben V. Pathak, Wendy Winslow, et al. "Glyphosate Infiltrates the Brain and Increases Pro-inflammatory Cytokine TNFα: Implications for Neurodegenerative Disorders," *Journal of Neuroinflammation,* vol. 19, no. 1 (July 28, 2022): p. 193.
9. Pere Puigbò, Lyydia I. Leino, Miia J. Rainio, et al. "Does Glyphosate Affect the Human Microbiota?" *Life,* vol. 12, no. 5 (May 9, 2022): p. 707.

Chapter 7: Psoriasis-Healing Foods

1. "Olijfoli Instituut," OliveOilInstitute.com (accessed January 22, 2026).

2. Elizabeth R. Mann, Ying Ka Lam, and Holm H. Uhlig. "Short-chain Fatty Acids: Linking Diet, the Microbiome and Immunity," *Nature Reviews: Immunology,* vol. 24, no. 8 (April 2, 2024): pp. 577–95.
3. Kate Dingwall. "Why Napa Green's Glyphosate Ban Is Such a Big Deal," *Wine Enthusiast* (December 7, 2023).
4. Wenjie Yang, Nahar Jannatun, Yanqiao Zeng, et al. "Impacts of Microplastics on Immunity," *Frontiers in Toxicology,* vol. 4 (September 27, 2022): 956885.

Chapter 8: The Healing Power of Your Mind

1. H.K. Beecher. "The Powerful Placebo," *Journal of the American Medical Association,* vol. 159, no17 (1955): pp. 1602–6.
2. Ted J. Kaptchuk, Elizabeth Friedlander, John M. Kelley, et al., "Placebos Without Deception: A Randomized Controlled Trial in Irritable Bowel Syndrome," PLoS One, vol. 5, no. 12 (December 22, 2010): p. e15591.
3. HeartMath Institute Research Staff. *Science of the Heart: Exploring the Role of the Heart in Human Performance* (Boulder Creek, CA.: HeartMath Institute, 2015).
4. Kanishk Chauhan, Alexander B. Neiman, and Peter A. Tass. "Synaptic Reorganization of Synchronized Neuronal Networks with Synaptic Weight and Structural Plasticity," *PLoS Computational Biology,* vol. 20, no. 7 (July 9, 2024): e1012261. Also *see,* Joanna Grover. "Your 2-Second Opportunity to Transform Negative Thinking," PsychologyToday.com (December 18, 2024).

5. "Walking in Beauty," VoxPopuliSphere.com (accessed March 17, 2026). This is an excerpt from the traditional closing prayer from the Navajo Blessing Way Ceremony. It honors the spiritual path of living in harmony within ourselves and with nature. The identity of the English translator is unknown to me.

Chapter 9: The Nontoxic Home and Self-Care

1. Scott Faber. "The Toxic Twelve Chemicals and Contaminants in Cosmetics," EWG.org (May 5, 2020).
2. Environmental Working Group. "What's in My Shaving Cream?" EWG.org (March 26, 2007).
3. Linfen Guo, Beilin Tu, Deng Li, et al. "Association Between United States Environmental Contaminants and the Prevalence of Psoriasis Derived from the National Health and Nutrition Examination Survey," *Toxics*, vol. 12, no. 7 (July 19, 2024): p. 522. Also *see*, Libby Schurr and Harriet Cheng. "Contact Allergy to Propylene Glycol," DermNetNZ.org (January 2022).
4. Sanne S. Meisser, Yasutaka Mitamura, Can Altunbulakli, et al. "Regulation of Immune Response Genes in the Skin of Allergic and Clinically Tolerant Individuals Exposed to p-Phenylenediamine," *Journal of Allergy*, vol. 79, no. 5 (May 2024): pp. 1291–305.
5. Irena Webb and Myrto Ashe. "What Is in Aveda Hair Color Ingredients?" IReadLabelsforYou.com (December 20, 2024).
6. Mayyadah S. Abed, Ahmed A. Moosa, and Mohammed A. Alzuhairi. "Heavy Metals in Cosmetics and Tattoos:

A Review of Historical Background, Health Impact, and Regulatory Limits," *Journal of Hazardous Materials Advances,* vol. 13 (February 2024): 100390.

7. Yang-Yiyi Yu, Hui Jin, and Qianjin Lu. "Effect of Polycyclic Aromatic Hydrocarbons on Immunity," *Journal of Translational Immunity,* vol. 5 (November 30, 2022): 100177.
8. Jeff Renaud. "Health Risks from Tattoo Inks not Just Skin Deep" MedicalXPress.com (July 12, 2021).
9. Artur Seweryn. "Interactions Between Surfactants and the Skin: Theory and Practice," *Advances in Colloid and Interface Science,* vol. 256 (June 2018): pp. 242–5. Also *see* Olusegun B. Samuel and Osaze V. Osayande. "Impact of Two Household Surfactants on Hepatic Lipid Peroxidation, Antioxidant Defense Responses and Hepatosomatic Index in Nile Tilapia, Oreochromis Niloticus," *Journal of Scientific Research and Development,* vol. 22, no. 1 (October 28, 2023): pp. 176–93.
10. "Showing All Products Containing Polyethylene Glycol" EWG's Guide to Healthy Cleaning, EWG.org (accessed January 23, 2026).
11. Priya Sellaturay, Shuaib Nasser, Sabita Islam, et. al. [Research Letter] "Polyethylene Glycol (PEG) Is a Cause of Anaphylaxis to the Pfizer/BioNTech mRNA COVID-19 Vaccine," *Clinical and Experimental Allergy,* vol. 51, no. 6 (June 2021): pp. 861–3.
12. Ying Zhang, Liang Lyu, Yue Tao, et al. "Health Risks of Phthalates: A Review of Immunotoxicity," *Environmental Pollution,* vol. 313 (November 15, 2022): 120173.

PART THREE: THE 90-DAY PSORIASIS-HEALING PROGRAM

Chapter 10: Three Months to Better Skin

1. Alexander V. Sorokin, Hildur Arnardottir, Maryia Svirydava, et al. "Comparison of the Dietary Omega-3 Fatty Acids Impact on Murine Psoriasis-like Skin Inflammation and Associated Lipid Dysfunction," *Journal of Nutritional Biochemistry,* vol. 117 (July 2023): 109348.
2. Ronald Prussick, Lisa Prussick, and Jimmy Gutman. "Psoriasis Improvement in Patients Using Glutathione-Enhancing, Nondenatured Whey Protein Isolate: A Pilot Study," *Journal of Clinical and Aesthetic Dermatology,* vol.6, no. 10 (Oct 2013): pp. 23–6.
3. Martyna Nowak-Perlak, Krzysztof Szpadel, Izabella Jabłońska, et al. "Promising Strategies in Plant-derived Treatments of Psoriasis: Update of In Vitro, In Vivo, and Clinical Trials Studies," *Molecules,* vol. 27, no. 3 (January 18, 2022): 591.
4. Jie Ma, Feifei Wang, Lei Wang, et al. "Inhibition of PI3K/AKT/GLUT1 Signaling Pathway by Quercetin in the Treatment of Psoriasis," *Frontiers in Bioscience,* vol. 30, no. 2 (2025): 26884.
5. Tara L. Whelan, J. Donald Dishman. et. al. "The Effect of Chiropractic Manipulation on Salivary Cortisol Levels,". *Journal of Manipulative Physiological Therapeutics,* vol 25, no. 3 (March–April 2002): pp. 149–53.
6. Dina Lelic, Imran Khan Niazi, Kelly Holt, et. al. "Manipulation of Dysfunctional Spinal Joints Affects Sensorimotor Integration in the Prefrontal Cortex: A

Brain Source Localization Study," *Journal of Neural Plasticity* (March 2016): article 3704964.

7. Imran Khan Niazi, Ernest Nlandu Kamavuako, et al. "The Effect of Spinal Manipulation on the Electrophysiological and Metabolic Properties of the Tibialis Anterior Muscle," *Journal of Healthcare,* vol. 8, no. 4 (December 10, 2020): p. 548.
8. Jeffrey J.W. Boyle, Nicholas Milne, Kevin P. Singer. "Influence of Age on Cervicothoracic Spinal Curvature: An Ex Vivo Radiographic Survey," *Clinical Biomechanics,* vol. 17, no. 5 (June 2022): pp. 361–7.
9. *Chiropractic and Consciousness: How We Influence Brain Plasticity.* Australian Spinal Research Foundation. (February 1, 2019).
10. David Ozeri. "Sleep Problems Common in Psoriasis," *Dermatology Times,* vol. 40, no. 9 (August 21, 2019).
11. American Heart Association. "How Much Sodium Should I Eat Per Day?" Heart.org (accessed March 30, 2026).
12. Sunny Lal. "Powerful Healing Benefits of Himalayan Salt Water," SelectSalt.com (accessed January 22, 2026).
13. Rhonda P. Patrick and Teresa L. Johnson. "Sauna Use as a Lifestyle Practice to Extend Healthspan," *Experimental Gerontology,* vol. 154 (October 15, 2021): 111509.

RESOURCES

Thank you for reading my book. If you are interested in pursuing additional resources or to connect with me, please visit my website AnikStMartin.com/skinonfire.

Anik St. Martin, D.C., DACCP
ADVANTAGE CHIROPRACTIC
1312 Vandercook Way
Longview, WA. 98632
Website: AnikStMartin.com
Telephone: (360) 425-6620

Mail-Order Products

FRESH-PRESSED OLIVE OIL
FreshPressedOliveOil.com

FOUR SIGMATIC MUSHROOM BLENDS
(powders you can add to coffee and smoothies)
For 20% off visit US.FourSigmatic.com/ANIK93919

DRY FARM WINES
DryFarmWines.com

BLUEBIRD GRAIN FARMS
(sustainable organic heirloom grains)
BluebirdGrainFarms.com

MOUNTAIN ROSE HERBS
(salt, herbs, teas, and body care products)
MountainRoseHerbs.com

CULTURES FOR HEALTH PRODUCTS
(cultured and fermented foods)
Culturesforhealth.com

BREADTOPIA: ARTISAN HOME BREAD BAKING
(sourdough and clean baking products)
Breadtopia.com

FINNISH SAUNA MANUFACTURER
(based in Portland, Oregon)
FinlandiaSaunas.com

GREEN VIBRANCE
(superfood supplement to implement daily)
VibrantHealth.com
For 20% off, use code myadvantagechiro

Organic Coffee Formulated for Health and Antioxidants

PURITY COFFEE
(my favorite)
For 20% off visit PurityCoffee.com/DRANIK

CLEAN COFFEE
CleanCoffeeCompany.com

BIODYNAMIC COFFEE
biodynamiccoffee.com

KION COFFEE
Kion.com

CSA and Farming Resources

COMMUNITY SUPPORTED AGRICULTURE COALITION
CSAcoalition.org

LOCAL HARVEST
LocalHarvest.org/CSA

Recommended Documentaries

Common Ground (2023), directed by Joshua Tickell and Rebecca Harrell Tickell

Fasting and the Longevity Revolution (2026), directed by Barry Alexander Brown

Food, Inc (2008), directed by Robert Kenner

Food, Inc. 2 (2023), directed by Robert Kenner and Melissa Robledo

Kiss the Ground (2020), directed by Joshua Tickell and Rebecca Harrell Tickell

The Biggest Little Farm (2018), directed by John Chester

To Which We Belong (2021), directed by Pamela Tanner Boll and Lindsay Richardson

Recommended Books

Autoimmune Paleo Cookbook: An Allergen-Free Approach to Managing Chronic Illness by Mickey Trescott

The Big Book of Kombucha: Brewing, Flavoring, and Enjoying the Health Benefits of Fermented Tea by Hannah Crum and Alex LaGory

The Divine Matrix: Bridging Time, Space, Miracles, and Belief by Gregg Braden

The Four Agreements: A Guide to Personal Freedom by Don Miguel Ruiz

Letting Go: The Pathway of Surrender by David R. Hawkins

Molecules of Emotion: The Science Behind Mind-Body Medicine by Candace B. Pert

The Naturally Clean Home, 3rd Edition: 150 Nontoxic Recipes for Cleaning and Disinfecting with Essential Oils by Karyn Siegel-Maier

Nourishing Traditions: The Cookbook That Challenges Politically Correct Nutrition and the Diet Dictocrats by Sally Fallon

The Power of Intention: Learning to Co-Create Your World Your Way by Wayne W. Dyer

The Secret by Rhonda Byrne

You Are the Placebo: Making Your Mind Matter by Joe Dispenza

The War of Art: Break Through the Blocks and Win Your Inner Creative Battles by Stephen Pressfield

Recommended Blogs

AutoimmuneWellness.com/blog
A great source for AIP recipes.

EWG.org
The Environmental Working Group is an organization that identifies the toxicity and safety of specific foods and lifestyle products.

HeartMath.org/research
The HeartMath Institute does heart-centered research.

Honest-Food.net
Recipes for foraging, wild game, fish, and fermenting.

PaleoRunningMomma.com
Easy paleo recipes.

RegenerativeFarmersofAmerica.com/blog
Info on how to find a farm or become a farmer.

ValterLongo.com
Information and recipes that will be useful for the Five-Day Fasting-Mimicking Cleanse.

ZachBushMD.com
A source of expertise on the microbiome, mindfulness, and other information.

ABOUT THE AUTHOR

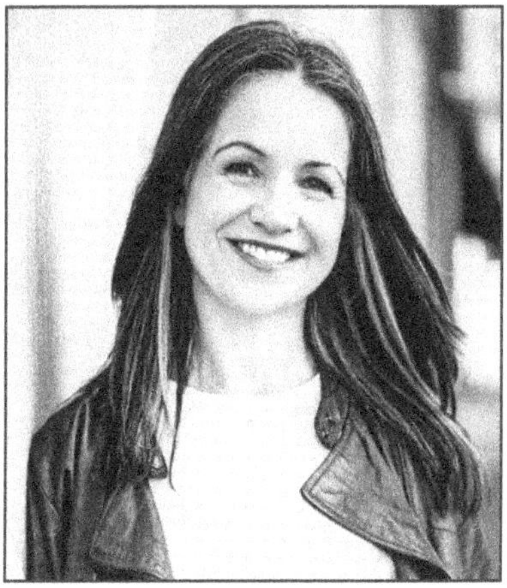

Anik St. Martin, D.C., DACCP, has owned and led a large holistic family wellness practice for twenty-five years. After a personal journey with autoimmunity and conducting over two decades of extensive research on psoriasis, Dr. St-Martin has developed, refined, and applied her expertise and experience to helping people of all ages overcome and cure their psoriasis.

Dr. St. Martin practices and lives with her husband, Dr. Darin Shook, in Washington State. When she isn't creating something in the kitchen, the couple spends their free time sailing and in the outdoors with their sons, Simon and Marco, and with their dogs, Stella and Charlotte.

www.ingramcontent.com/pod-product-compliance
Lightning Source LLC
LaVergne TN
LVHW022203200926
848481LV00006B/1833